Your Hormones in Harmony

⇒ A Smart Woman's Guide
To a Lifetime of Energy, Focus, and Vitality ⇐

by
Dr. Melodie M. Billiot

Published by
Wellness Ink

Your Hormones in Harmony: A Smart Woman's Guide to a Lifetime of Energy, Focus, and Vitality, by Dr. Melodie M. Billiot

Evectics is a service mark owned by Dr. Melodie M. Billiot.

For more information, contact:

Dr. Melodie M. Billiot
Alternative Health Atlanta
1640 Powers Ferry Rd.
Building 14 Suite 100
Marietta, GA 30067
770-937-9200

Email: DrMBilliot@AlternativeHealthAtlanta.com

Website: www.AlternativeHealthAtlanta.com

ISBN: 978-1-988645-16-2 (digital)

ISBN: 978-1-988645-15-5 (print)

Attention: Quantity discounts and customized versions are available for bulk purchases. For permission requests or quantity discounts, please email Dr. Billiot at DrMBilliot@AlternativeHealthAtlanta.com

Cover design: Archangel Ink

Original cover art by Lynda Goldman

Printed in the United States

Disclaimer

The information in this book is designed to provide helpful information on the subjects discussed. This book is not meant to be used, nor should it be used, to diagnose or treat any medical condition. For diagnosis or treatment of any medical problem, consult your own physician. The publisher and author are not responsible for any specific health needs or conditions that may require medical supervision and are not liable for any damages or negative consequences from any treatment, action, application or preparation, to any person reading or following the information in this book. References are provided for informational purposes only and do not constitute endorsement of any websites or other sources. Readers should be aware that the websites listed in this book may change.

Gifts for You

I wrote *Your Hormones in Harmony* to start you on the road to resolving your health problems and living a lifestyle that prevents them from ever reoccurring.

Here are two gifts from me personally to continue your progress:

Free book: *Get Your Life Back*. This is a short, hard-hitting, practical "how-to" for anyone with an unresolving health condition. Recovering from a chronic health condition requires knowledge and the right attitude. This book can help with both!

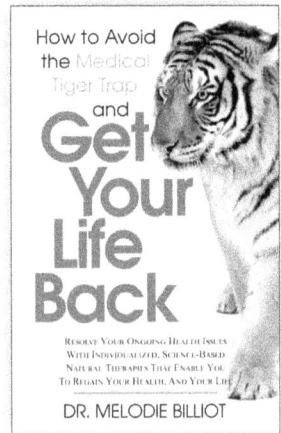

How to Avoid the Medical Tiger Trap and **Get Your Life Back**

RESOLVE YOUR ONGOING HEALTH ISSUES WITH INDIVIDUALIZED, SCIENCE-BASED NATURAL THERAPIES THAT ENABLE YOU TO REGAIN YOUR HEALTH, AND YOUR LIFE

DR. MELODIE BILLIOT

Free course: *Xenoestrogens and Endocrine Disruptors.* You may have never heard these words before, but if you have a hormone problem, chances are they are heavily involved. These are the environmental toxins that most affect your hormones. They are in your food, water, drugs, makeup and personal products. Understanding what these compounds are and how they disrupt your hormones is a key part of recovering and keeping your health.

The course lessons are delivered by email and help you to fully understand this "un-understandable" subject. It took delivering over 400 public lectures on endocrine disruptors for me to finally work out a simple, fun way to teach the subject.

To get these and other free resources, scan the QR code below, or visit AlternativeHealthAtlanta.com/HarmonyGifts. Enjoy!

– Dr. Billiot

Praise for *Your Hormones in Harmony*

If you want to heal your body and regain your vitality, follow the wisdom in this book very carefully!

As a nurse practitioner and integrative/functional health coach, I've worked with many bright, talented, health care providers. In my career of over thirty-five years, I've never met anyone who is more brilliant about health and healing than Dr. Melodie Billiot. As a busy professional woman whose health crashed after trying to "do it all" for way too many years, I was often told, "It's all in your head," and, "There's nothing wrong with you."

It was Dr. Billiot's care, compassion and expertise that helped me make vitality my reality again. If you want to heal your body and regain your vitality, follow the wisdom in this book very carefully!

– Lori Finlay Hamilton
MS, RN, APRN (RT), BCC

This book has the most important and correct information about hormone health. It is the place to start for any woman who has questions about her hormones.

Dr. Billiot shows you that your hormone problems are not just from stress, not just from toxins, not just age, and not just lack of exercise; and although these problems may be common, they are not normal. It doesn't have to be this way!

I read this book to write a review and found myself learning a whole lot in the process! *Your Hormones in Harmony* is a very well thought-out and complete account of how your hormones got so out of balance, and into a downward spiral. This book will show you how to return the dynamics of your hormone system to balance and harmony.

– Dr. Stewart Edrich DC
Applied Kinesiologist, Holistic Health Solutions, Los Alamitos, CA

Dr. Billiot has produced a remarkably simple and practical book which portends an innovative and important approach to women's health.

There is little doubt that the increased number of manmade, xenoestrogenic compounds we find in water, air, food and household products can disrupt normal hormonal functions. As a potent example, these chemicals have been linked to an increase in breast cancer over the past fifty years at almost a pandemic rate. In this book, Your Hormones in Harmony, Dr. Billiot's patient narratives bring a decidedly real, human touch to a subject that is all too often cold, diagnostic jargon.

– Michael Wisner
Research Scientist and Author of Living Healthy in a Toxic World

First, *Your Hormones in Harmony* is written by a woman; a trained, skillful, healthcare professional who cares about women and the quality of life we can have.

Second, it is readable, and offers to assist us in making well-informed decisions regarding our health and welfare.

Last, my life is one of living proof that if you accept any or all of what Dr. Billiot offers us in this work there is no question that proportionately you will improve upon where you were before you became enlightened.

– Yvette Cologne,
Executive-Level Government Administrator, Georgia

Dr. Billiot writes with passion, and a vision for a healthier tomorrow for all women!

Her book, *Your Hormones in Harmony*, is not only insightful and educational but also very understandable. She lays out the roles of hormones and how they affect our wellbeing in a clear and concise manner.

Dr. Billiot shares the story of her own personal health and journey towards a balanced life. Through her work, Dr. Billiot deepens our understanding of what we encounter as women in everyday life, and the factors that can wreak havoc on our hormonal system. Overall, Dr. Billiot's book is filled with understanding, awareness and inspiration as she brings us full circle on the pathway to hormone harmony!

– Stephanie Clement
RYT, CSYT, MT, CYT, owner of Stillness Yoga & Meditation Center

Dr. Billiot puts forth in a candid, understandable, appealing and personal way an explanation of many common women's issues that are often just as commonly misunderstood.

Fifteen years of providing medical thermographic services to thousands of women has allowed me the unique opportunity to witness which methods and modalities of treatment benefit the patient the most. I also hear from the ladies I image of their frustrations with our current healthcare options, and how confusing those can be.

Just as thermography isn't just for breasts, there is a lot more to the hormone system than the five or six sex hormones most doctors concern themselves with. True remedies and health solutions require addressing the entire body as a whole. This book offers many holistic options and lots of encouragement!

Only you can begin to make the changes necessary for your own health, and you have lots of help in *Your Hormones in Harmony*!

"Be fierce! Be beautiful! Be you!"

– Nina Rea
BCTT, PhysioTherms, Inc.

"This book is a MUST READ for every man and woman!"

Your Hormones in Harmony is the doorway to every woman's vibrant health. Dr. Billiot walks us through that doorway with clear, simple explanations that address the causes of misery and ill health in almost every woman.

The best part is that she explains everything in a very simple, easy-to-understand language that everyone can relate to. I felt that she took me on a journey from my teens to my golden years, explaining the role of my hormones through every phase of my life.

This book is an easy and interesting read because of the wit and humor that Dr. Billiot uses to lighten up medical explanations that are so often very dry to read.

With the valuable information in this book, women can understand what is happening to their bodies and why, and as a result, be more capable of taking care of them. Men will realize why their wives, mothers, sisters and daughters are at one moment, Antheia, Goddess of Flowers, and at the next, Hekate, Goddess of the Night. Their loved ones are not crazy, only a victim of out-of-balance hormones!

The clear and comprehensive program in this book fits perfectly with holistic, empirical and time-tested nutritional and natural methods for avoiding medical pitfalls and bringing back the symphony and homeostasis of the body to sustain a blissful life.

– Nelli Biddix
ND, CBS, CHS, ACNC, MH

I love the theme "knowledge is power." This book is exactly that, a powerful tool in the hands of those seeking to regain their health.

It addresses topics that no one else is willing to discuss, and provides much needed guidance to healthy living in a world of profit-driven companies selling lies to an unassuming public. A must-read for anyone desiring to live a healthy and happy lifestyle!

– Aubrey Van Benthem
Author and Teacher

"If you are interested and concerned about women's health issues, especially your breasts, this book is for you!"

My favorite chapter is about taking charge of your body and health and not depending on a doctor to decide for you. Doctors should partner with you, which is often not the case in conventional medicine.

Dr. Billiot's book is informative, easy to read and easy to understand. It covers hormone information, lab testing, the effects of stress on our body, female health disorders, and care options. Most importantly, *Your Hormones in Harmony* tells you how to have a lifetime of ENERGY, FOCUS, VITALITY, and more!

As an RN of fifty years, a holistic nurse practitioner, a licensed massage therapist specializing in cancer and mastectomy, and a breast health educator, I am truly impressed about the quality of information this book provides. As much as I thought I was a wealth of knowledge, Dr. Billiot's book provided me with wonderful new information! A great read for all women regardless of age!

– Cheryl Chapman
RN, BSN, HN-BC, LMT, NCBTMB

Dedication

I lovingly dedicate this book to my wonderful husband and amazing sons.

To my husband Norman who loves and supports me no matter what. He is truly the wind beneath my wings. I am so grateful for his love and never-ending optimism in our life and in our business together of helping others find health. He is the motivation and the energy for all of us.

To my precious sons Alec and Drew, without you I would be a shadow of who I am today. Being a mother to two amazing sons can do that for you! To Alec, my artist, you are an inspiration, and as a result of our journey together to find your health answers, we have helped thousands. You are a blessing to me and to many others in this world. To Drew, you have been my light and encouragement and my sunbeam every day since you came to us. You keep me young, and you always make me laugh. You will be a force in this world! I can't imagine life without either of you!

EDITORIAL NOTE: Informational links are provided throughout this book, primarily in footnotes.

Readers should be aware that these links are subject to change. For a full list of clickable links referenced here, visit:

www.AlternativeHealthAtlanta.com/Harmony

Contents

§ **CHAPTER 14**
Now It's Up to You: Take Charge and Take Action! 171

§ **CHAPTER 15**
Women Who Took Charge of Their Health 177

Foreword

Dr. Melodie Billiot has written a much-needed book that I believe is a "must read" for all women. It's a smart and insightful discussion about the struggles that most women will face at one point or another in their life.

This book explains clearly and simply the causes of our most common and frustrating problems with our body and mind. While it is great to have affirmation for why you feel the way you do, having a path of correction is much more important! So many women do not understand their bodies or how they work and have spent a lifetime of having them manipulated by drugs or worse, surgery. Women need information to feel empowered about the decisions they will make about their body. And most importantly, they need that information before they find themselves in a serious health crisis!

Dr. Billiot covers the basics behind female physiology and how it changes during all the stages in your life. She discusses the unique challenges women face— and those many things that can disrupt the natural balance of hormones, such as the millions of women put on birth control pills to "regulate" their period instead of correcting the underlying imbalance. Exposure to this drug may be just the beginning of a hormone disruption that can create a cascade of metabolic issues, all to be treated with more medication!

Dr. Billiot shows women the choices they have and outlines what they need to do to be truly healthy. She talks about getting to the root cause, the "why" behind their current state of health and setting them on a path they can follow for a lifetime. I have seen many books and many other doctors promising to do this. Most don't succeed, and many make suggestions that end up being harmful down the road. She and I have both worked in this field for many years… and we are all too familiar with the messes we have been left to clean up from patients who have taken bad advice. This book could make the difference for so many women to avoid their becoming "another mess" to be cleaned up (if they are lucky enough to find a doctor who knows how to do this). Dr. Billiot takes us far beyond symptom chasing and mere symptom relief.

I often say, "Patients don't know what they don't know," but if they could understand their bodies and their health better, they would make a more informed decision. There has been too much cover-up of symptoms in our health care system and it's past time for a change. Dr. Billiot has done a beautiful job teaching women what they need to know about their bodies and their health.

On a personal note, I have known Dr. Billiot for years. She's an incredibly intelligent, hardworking and caring doctor. She has helped so many women already! My hope is that her book will empower even more women to be more proactive about their health. If you have picked this book up in hopes of finding some answers and maybe to have some hope, you won't be disappointed. I think every woman could benefit from reading this book. It would also be a good read for all health care practitioners who are involved with women's health. We are all here to learn, teach and grow!

– Annette Kutz Schippel, DC,
Endocrine Wellness, LLC

Preface

This book is for the sick, exhausted woman I was twenty-five years ago, after I finished graduate school. It is for all the women, who, like the younger me, wake up in the morning exhausted and stay that way all day. This book is for the ladies who have worked themselves almost to death in high school and college, at work and as a mom or business woman.

It is for all the women trying to live up to the expectations others set for them and the unrealistic ones they set for themselves. This book is for the lovely women who come to my practice on an increasing basis, mentally and physically depleted and sometimes chemically dependent on drugs and chemicals to survive.

It is not a pretty picture. These women are our future. They are the moms of our current and next generations and they are sicker and sadder and facing more challenges than ever before in a currently very unforgiving job market and economy.

Statistics show that millennial women experience depression 15.7 more days per year than their male counterparts. Illness, disability and overall poor health make it difficult for women to thrive at home and in the workplace. The Institute for Women's Policy Research analysis indicates that women ages eighteen and older who participated in the CDC's 2013 Behavioral Risk Factor Surveillance System survey, reported that their activities were limited by their health status for an average of 4.8 days in the month preceding the survey.

Women and mothers are the backbone of our world and they need help now. Health issues that begin at a young age will very often result in long term chronic disease later on.

This book will tell you why this is happening to you. What you do not know will hurt you in this case. You will learn that it isn't your fault that you cannot perform as you would like to and why you feel so exhausted all the time. You will receive answers to why your body and mind seem to be failing you and what to do about it naturally and without drugs.

Find out how to live a vibrant and joyful life, how to have a balanced life and balanced hormones. Every phase of your life is the best time of your life! We all have our futures in front of us! Don't live that future trapped by exhaustion, anxiety and fear. Get your life and your health back, now and for your future!

– Dr. Melodie Billiot
Founder of Alternative Health Atlanta
Marietta, GA
April 2018

Harmony is pure love,
for love is a concerto.
— Lope de Vega

CHAPTER 1
Stop the Madness!

If hormone problems have ever made you ill, you know the madness I'm talking about. If you have ever been sad for so many reasons and for no reason at all, you understand the madness. If you are a young girl or woman troubled by extremely painful periods, missing hours or days of your life in a haze of pain and pain killers, you know the madness. If you have hot flashes and night sweats, feeling heat rising off your body during that meeting at work or waking up soaking wet and having to change your pajamas and sheets, you know about the madness. If you suffer from chronic skin problems and food allergies, or intolerances that cause stomach pain and nausea or other discomforts every time you eat, you know about the madness. If you have ever become very angry at the drop of a hat and screamed at those you love and then later, with much shame and regret, realized it was really a trivial matter, then you too understand this madness. Insomnia, exhaustion, mood changes, constant weight gain, depression, and anxiety are all part of the madness.

The madness is often connected to our hormones. Those little microscopic amounts of substance can give us the time of our lives or make a ruin of them.

What are these things called hormones? How do they run us the way they do? How can we have more control over them?

I have been in practice as a chiropractor and holistic doctor using clinical nutrition, herbs, Chinese medicine and functional medicine for 24 years. I have seen kids grow up and go to college. Some of my favorite patients have grown old in good health while others have left this world in a very difficult fashion, often as a result of their life choices. I have heard many stories and had the honor and privilege of sharing in many lives.

I have long wanted to write a book about how to live a healthy life throughout your whole life. I decided to do it now because too many people are suffering, too many people are looking for answers to their health problems and are being met with myths and misinformation and outright lies.

As a woman, I have been privileged to live through several hormone cycles of life; as a wellness specialist, I have seen patients live through them too. Each stage offers a unique window of growth for us as human beings and as women.

Hormones and the menstrual cycle

Adolescence is often a very unstable and difficult stage of life. Women's menstrual cycles are far from uniform.[*]

The beginning of this female cycle is for many the start of a life of stress, pain, depression or worse. Over the course of my practice I have seen many women begin their adult lives with hormone imbalance and other health issues that have never been resolved and have only worsened over time— sometimes for life, because of the very solutions they have been offered. Most of these early onset conditions, and their underlying concerns, were never diagnosed correctly. These young women have either been offered no solutions or solutions that include the birth control pill to "regulate" their cycle, or anti-depressants to "fix" their moods. Women come to me in their forties and fifties on anti-depressants and anti-anxiety meds, which they've been taking since their teen years. As a result, they have been unable to stop using them because the root cause of their hormonal imbalance or other health condition was never found.

The young girl who was once miserable with a flooding cycle and horrible cramps is now a nervous, anxious woman in her thirties or forties, exhausted and stressed, possibly diagnosed with thyroid nodules, Polycystic Ovarian Syndrome[**] or other hormonal conditions. This woman is likely taking antidepressants and has often turned to other drugs and chemicals to survive. She may smoke marijuana or drink wine at night to sleep and then drink copious amounts of coffee or take caffeine pills or drink energy drinks to be able to get through her busy schedule.

Or, as one of my patients described it, she had to "Elvis it" to keep going. To her, that meant alcohol at night to sleep and caffeine all day to stay awake. This woman was in graduate school trying to keep pace with her school

---

[*] www.ncbi.nlm.nih.gov/pubmed/122422

[**] *PCOS is a condition of increased testosterone, producing male pattern hair growth on the face and body, often accompanied by ovarian cysts, insulin resistance and irregular, or absent, menstrual cycles and sometimes infertility issues.*

work and not understanding her exhaustion. She expressed dismay at how her body seemed to betray her when she needed it the most.

Often women in their thirties have young children and are exhausted by work and home responsibilities. These women also know that if they don't get it all done no one else will. The child rearing phase of life can be challenging, and many of the women I meet do not know there is help available. It is not normal to feel completely wrung dry all the time—this should be the time of your life!

The beginnings of more serious health issues have already taken root by the time you reach your thirties and forties. By now you may have struggled for years with nagging health concerns, doing your best to self-medicate or trying to ignore your growing health issues.

I recently met with a dear patient who was obviously suffering from many health issues, but the only thing she would write on her entry form was "occasional back pain". She had spent years telling herself that she was fine, ignoring many health issues as they developed—after all, how can you acknowledge you are sick when you have so much to do? She had an extremely busy schedule, managing her family and a full-time job in a male-dominated field. For her to admit that she was not perfect, that she was somehow lacking, was more than she could easily handle.

It was very hard for her to see that she was not as good or perfect as she had pretended for so many years. Admitting that she did not have the good health she imagined felt like a personal betrayal! After all, she'd lived for years making it all work, doing it all and being a super woman. Now she was pre-diabetic, exhausted, on three blood pressure meds and still pushing herself to be the best she thought she could be. It was time for this sweet woman to love herself and be honest about her health for the first time in her life.

For many of us, this is the first step we must take, to realize that something is wrong. Once we can do this, something can be done about the problems.

By the time they reach their fifties or sixties, many women have had a hysterectomy because of fibroids or continued heavy menstrual flow, leading their doctors to determine that their female parts are no longer useful and should be removed! Women are told they are in menopause now and do not really need these organs any more, or other such questionable logic. This often leads to synthetic hormone replacement therapy, which carries its own health risks and complications. For some women, this time of life can be fraught with ill health. It is not uncommon for someone to be prescribed two or three blood pressure meds and possibly a statin drug for high cholesterol along with an anti-depressant or anti-anxiety drug.

This same woman could be battling pre-diabetes, high blood pressure or a full-blown case of diabetes, with stubborn weight that now won't ever let go. She is often exhausted, hot flashing, experiencing insomnia and facing even more serious health issues like osteoporosis and heart disease, often because of unbalanced or deficient female hormones.

Look at these top 10 clues that you may have entered this cycle of ill health and are headed down the wrong path. If you see yourself in any of these, your health may need serious attention. How many of these symptoms do you have right now?

1. Your symptoms get in the way of your life: pain, fatigue, insomnia, brain fog, depression, menstrual and menopause problems, allergies, irritability, weight gain, anxiety, gas, bloating, reflux, indigestion, constipation, diarrhea, breathing problems, low immune response, rashes, joint pain, vision and hearing problems, itchy skin, hair loss, acne, back pain, neck pain, headaches, infertility, low libido, trouble concentrating, memory problems, sugar cravings, bone loss, blood sugar problems, high blood pressure, fibroid tumors, heart problems, high cholesterol and more.

2. Doctors give you treatments that don't help these symptoms or fix the underlying problems and leave you angry and frustrated.

3. Doctors or others say or imply that there's really nothing wrong with you. Maybe "it's all in your head". They tell you you're getting all the treatment available so why are you still whining? This despite your obvious and serious symptoms and health problems.

4. You feel your spouse, boss, coworkers and friends have no clue that you just aren't functioning normally a lot of the time.

5. You feel frustration, disappointment and guilt that you can't keep up with everything. Or you are paying a physical and mental price just to do the minimum required in your life.

6. You are upset by the money you have wasted in co-pays, uninsured medical treatment and drugs, all those therapies and the fifty bottles of vitamins on your shelf that didn't help.

7. You sometimes feel as if your life is being stolen—with periods of time you aren't fully "there", and lost times with family and friends that you've had to turn down because you just weren't up to it.

8. You are confused by all the conflicting information on the Internet and in books about why you have these problems and what will make them go away. You feel frustration at all the "other people" who say these things helped them—when they aren't helping you.

9. You have a recurring fear that you will never find a solution and that the rest of your life is going to be this way.

10. You have a recurring fear that all this suffering is going to get a lot worse in the future.

Chronic health conditions— a silent and terrifying epidemic

According to the Centers for Disease Control and Prevention (CDC), "As of 2012, about half of all adults in America—117 million people—had one or more chronic health conditions. One in four adults had two or more chronic health conditions. Seven of the top ten causes of death in 2014 were chronic diseases. Two of these chronic diseases—heart disease and cancer—together accounted for nearly 46% of all deaths."

Those statistics are terrifying. When we examine that list of "clues" that help us identify health issues, most of those symptoms are chronic health conditions with a lifestyle component that we can control! The problem is that most people do not know their bodies can heal and get better, and that they can achieve a higher level of health for themselves.

So, when a patient feels she must "go the medical route," I really do understand. Of course, some problems truly are medical problems. These issues can be expected to resolve with medical treatment, and the side effects of the treatment are acceptable. Broken bones, severe infections and diseases, requiring body systems support, all fall into this category.

But the average person has absolutely no idea what can be accomplished with modern alternative health technology, working with the body to help it to heal. In fact, most are not even looking for non-medical solutions.

This is because there is a very important fact they haven't yet discovered: There are few-to-no effective medical treatments for chronic health problems—and almost no one is talking about this.

In fact, the most common way people discover this fact is when their doctor says, "There is nothing more that can be done for you." You developed a health complaint and dutifully went to your doctor to have it fixed—with no idea there would be a problem. Then, suddenly, you were stuck with a health condition that seemingly had no solution.

This is like a tiger trap—a camouflaged hole covered over with grass that you don't see until after you have fallen into it.

Chronic health problems are those that recur regularly or never go away. They make up a huge majority of all health problems, costing 75 cents of every healthcare dollar. The gaping hole in modern health care is that there are almost no solutions for these problems, only drug management to make the symptoms somewhat more tolerable. This massive deficiency is not discussed or pointed out publicly; indeed, you may be completely unaware of it—until you develop this type of problem yourself.

Before you developed a chronic condition, chances are you had the same ideas most of the unaffected population does:

"What's a chronic health condition?"

"If you are sick, just go to the doctor—what's the big deal?"

This is reflected in the media's reporting on health care, which consists of politics, business, and medical and drug studies that make the news and current events. Nowhere is it pointed out that nearly half of the public reading the news has a health problem with no effective treatment available.

What the media and public don't see is the individual suffering of those with long-term health conditions, which reduces happiness and productivity for them and their families. These are not the severely ill who are bedridden, living on disability or requiring constant care. For the most part, they are people who hold down jobs, take care of their families, raise children and are active in churches, synagogues and other civic and social organizations.

But every day they wonder if they can keep it up. They're battling fatigue, depression, pain, brain fog and the conviction that it's all likely to get worse. They believe this because over many years of research and effort, they have found no effective treatments or solutions. These people have found that medical technology is very close to bankrupt on the subject of chronic illness and offers nothing other than temporary or long-term drug management of symptoms as solutions.

"You are healthy, congratulations!"

The nature of many chronic health problems is that sometimes they don't show as out of range on blood tests, or as anything of concern, during a standard physical. The person will complain of many symptoms to their doctor, but the doctor may tell them, after labs and examination, that they are perfectly healthy. They may be told to reduce their stress, eat less fat and get more rest, but there is no diagnosis. Often if the person continues to insist that there is something wrong, the doctor will suggest, "It's possibly depression or a 'stress-related' issue,"—implying that if the doctor fails to find the problem, it must be because the patient is making it up or it is a mentally induced problem on the part of the patient. Often patients are prescribed an anti-depressant or other psychotropic drug.

Just as one example, according to the CDC arthritis causes more than 22 million Americans to have trouble with their usual activities. Modern medicine has no cure for arthritis and can only "manage" it as long as possible with drugs—all with severe side effects. Further, there is no arthritis case that is only arthritis. This is a condition of chronic inflammation which creates a host of other chronic health problems to go along with the debilitating joint pain.

Below are some of the side effects of arthritis drugs.

- **NSAIDS (non-steroidal anti-inflammatories)** Blood clots, heart attack, stroke.
- **STEROIDS** Cataracts, bone loss, increased blood sugar and appetite.
- **DMARDs (disease modifying anti-rheumatic drug)** Increased susceptibility to infection.
- **BIOLOGICS** Increased risk of serious infections.

If you have fallen into this camouflaged hole, this tiger trap, don't be fooled into imagining that anyone is coming to your rescue.

There are no miracle cures right around the corner because the health care system is completely stuck on the drug treatment model, which does not work for most chronic problems.

David Shaywitz, a healthcare reporter writing in Forbes magazine, inadvertently got it right. In an article defending the pharmaceutical industry from charges of withholding cures they don't want you to know about he writes:

> *The unfortunate truth is that drug companies really want to cure disease, but rarely know how. Medical science simply isn't up to the challenge. Most diseases aren't well enough understood to enable the rational development of truly transformative treatments.*

Of course, by "treatments" Mr. Shaywitz means drugs. A drug is a chemical that forces the body to react, not a resource that the body can use to heal itself of a chronic problem. There may be no conspiracy to keep the cure for your problems hidden, but the truth is just as bad: most of the research being done to treat chronic problems is in the area of drugs, which are not, and never have been an effective solution.

To sum up

There is a class of health problems that can ruin (or is currently ruining) your health, life and happiness, and it affects at least 50% of the U.S. population.

Little-to-no effective medical treatment is available if this happens to you or your family.

There is little understanding or empathy for these sufferers, as most of the world seems to believe that doctors know how to treat all but the big-name diseases (like cancer, MS, Alzheimer's, etc.) quite effectively. If you are suffering from other than a big-name disease and are complaining about it, the popular thinking is that you need to go get treatment and, frankly, suck it up. You don't have a real problem. In some cases, this attitude may be shared by your doctor.

This is the useless cycle of chronic pain and chronic illness that I want to help you prevent. If you see yourself in any of these clues or in any of these chronic illnesses, you can do something about it now, and the fact that you are reading this book is a good start.

The women I help are the movers and shakers, the ambitious goal-oriented women who are here on this earth to make a difference. They have children to raise, jobs to do, movies to make, books to write and people to help all over this world. My patients are mothers, and wives, CEOs, CFOs, nurses, doctors, and teachers, hair dressers, sales reps, flight attendants, artists, entrepreneurs. They are the makers and the creators, the starters of charities and non-profits that serve those in need. They are IT and project managers, students, actresses and stunt people. They are musicians and lawyers and accountants and school counselors. They are the person you see in the mirror every morning. They are you. They have too much to do and accomplish to be sick and tired. And they know their health is worth the time the effort and the money that it may take to get to wellness. They are not afraid. They are amazing. They are strength. They are my heroes!

These years should be the times of our lives, but for many of us they are not. Come with me on a journey to meet some of these women who are perhaps just like you. Come and see what can be done for you so that you can have the time of your life—for *all* your life!

CHAPTER 2

Your Beautiful Hormones and How They Make You YOU!

The more you understand your own body the better advocate you will be for yourself and your health, so in that light, let's examine the menstrual cycle. It's a complicated system, made beautiful by the harmony of the many hormones that make it work.

To examine the menstrual cycle is to examine the beautiful harmony of our hormones. For many women, there is a mystery that sometimes creates a fear of what's "down there" and how it all works. The dark and sometimes mysterious parts of your beautiful body need to be understood.

I want you to understand how your body works, what parts do what, why your hormones do the things they sometimes do, and when and how you can get pregnant. If you know these things, it may possibly shine some light on why you haven't yet been able to achieve pregnancy and why your body is doing what it is doing.

Much has been written about the female body, and there are too many nicknames and too much incorrect and negative information written and spoken about our beautiful bodies for me to even mention—so I won't.

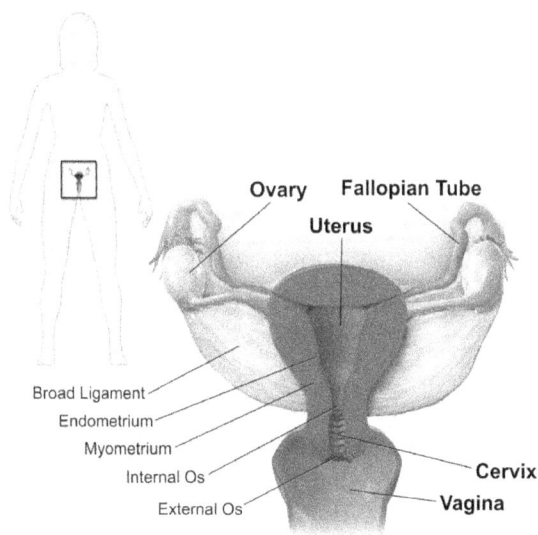

I am going to tell you the simple truth. We will use the correct names of body parts and learn the function of each one. Knowledge is power, and on this subject, it can be very powerful indeed as you can use it to manage not only your health but that of your family as well.

So, without further ado, I'd like you to meet your hormones! I will define what a hormone is and then look at each of the major hormones in our cycle, as well as the basic anatomy of the female body.

According to the Merriam-Webster online dictionary, a hormone is "any of various chemical substances produced by body cells and released especially into the blood and having a specific effect on cells or organs of the body usually at a distance from the place of origin." The major female hormones you should know are estrogen, progesterone, testosterone, luteinizing hormone and follicle stimulating hormone. This team is responsible for the regulation of your menstrual cycle, which is in turn responsible for your fertility and many other health aspects of your body.

Your hormones are amazing substances! They are your body's messengers and have a very strong influence on all your organs. When they are at their best, these hormones somehow all coordinate and work together to create a symphony of magic in your body!

My favorite class in university was endocrinology, or the study of hormones. It was a miracle and a wonder to me as I studied this system that such important effects came from such tiny messengers, and that somehow the cascades of hormones streaming through the body had meaning. They all seemed to follow the same conductor to produce their music. As you might imagine, of course, when those hormones become unbalanced that symphony is going to be very much out of tune! In my opinion, the beauty and complexity of our hormone system is unmatched.

Have you ever wondered what a hormone is made of? Cholesterol!! Crazy, right? Who would have thought that!

Do you know what makes your hormonal orchestra play beautifully all the time? Nutrients, and lots of them!

The endocrine system (or hormone system) is impacted severely by nutritional imbalances and deficiencies. Making and replacing our hormones daily requires many different nutrients, and most of us are not getting these nutrients from our diets. You truly are what you eat! All your physical functions require nutrients, and your female hormones need many of these!

Picture your hormones as double-ended keys. The receptor end fits into the cell and "unlocks" the door to start an action. The other end fits exactly with other enzymes that can transform the hormone into another hormone or target it to be let go from the body.[*]

The beautiful symphony that is the female cycle

Your female cycle is magic. It's what creates new life on earth. We women hold the seed of creation inside our bodies! What an honor to hold in your own physical self the future generations of earth! Helping young girls understand this honor should be a priority as we nurture strong and independent women.

Understanding from this perspective can give girls and young women respect for their bodies, and ultimately for themselves. Viewing our female bodies in a derogatory and demeaning manner is a dishonor and a disgrace to all sexes. Sex and the reproduction of the body are beautiful things. This beauty has been stolen by the coarse and the fearfully misinformed, and subverted to a dark and sometimes dirty and evil subject.

Sex and reproduction have been subjected to many thousands of years of social and religious taboos, and many books have been written on the topic. It has been, and will continue to be, a difficult subject for the societies of earth. Suffice it to say that the basic purpose of sex includes both reproduction and the resulting pleasure for those involved. The female menstruation cycle, and the gestation cycle that results in a new human being, are nothing short of a miracle—a beautiful symphony of hormones in harmony and balance.

The phases of the cycle

Here's a link to a YouTube video by Glamour magazine, which in two minutes describes your cycle and your possible moods during this time. youtube.com/watch?v=WOi2Bwvp6hw

---

[*] *Jonathon Wright MD, and John Morgenthaler, Natural Hormone Replacement For Women Over 45 (1997)*

The female cycle has several phases, when your major hormones go up and down throughout the month causing ovulation and menstruation.

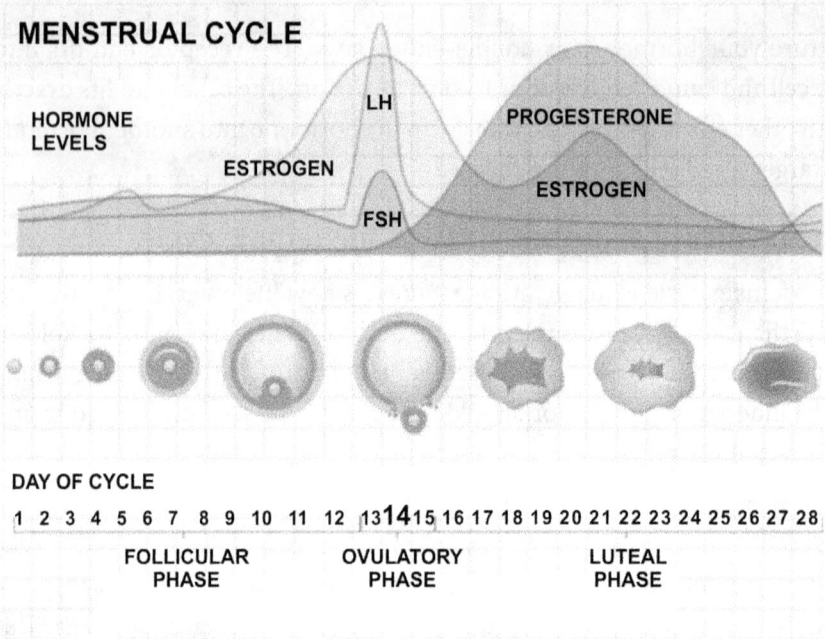

MENSTRUAL CYCLE

HORMONE LEVELS

LH

ESTROGEN

FSH

PROGESTERONE

ESTROGEN

DAY OF CYCLE

1 2 3 4 5 6 7 8 9 10 11 12 13 14 15 16 17 18 19 20 21 22 23 24 25 26 27 28

FOLLICULAR PHASE   OVULATORY PHASE   LUTEAL PHASE

Day 1 of your cycle is the first day you begin bleeding. It is not the light spotting that happens sometimes a few days before-hand. Sometimes a woman may "spot" for a day or two very lightly before menstruation begins. Day 1 is the first day of the true cycle or when the blood begins to flow. This beginning day of your menstruation is used to calculate approximate ovulation and the start of your next menses. It is important to know this date to accurately predict your pregnancy due date.

You could spend hours studying this extremely important body process. Here is a basic overview of your menstrual cycle.

The Follicular Phase is the first part of your cycle and is run mainly by estrogen. An average female bleeds for about 3–7 days; some more, some less. The first part of the cycle is about building up the uterine lining for a possible pregnancy. This is when ovulation occurs, at about Day 14 for a woman with a 28-day cycle. Many amazing things happen during this time to prepare the body for pregnancy, and besides planning for a pregnancy, this information can be used to assist with birth control.

The second phase of the menstrual cycle is called the **Luteal Phase**, and is run by the progesterone hormone. During this part of the cycle, your hormones will cause a ripening of the uterine lining in preparation for possible pregnancy and will help the body keep the embryo safe if implantation occurs. This phase, when working correctly, helps prevent spontaneous abortions and ensures a smooth menstruation.

When no pregnancy occurs, both estrogen and progesterone fall, signaling the start of another cycle, and bleeding begins again. If pregnancy does occur, the embryo produces small amounts of hormones that communicate the need for more progesterone. The hormones LH (luteinizing hormone) and FSH (follicle stimulating hormone) are important in the maturing of the egg follicle and to trigger ovulation.

LH and FSH work in concert with estrogen and progesterone and come from the brain, not the ovaries or other female organs. Observe the perfection of these hormones working together to create the few days out of the month that the body can reproduce.

The organs secrete certain hormones that communicate in various ways with other parts of the body. These organs then secrete their own hormones in response, and—wonder of all wonders—if these hormones and organs harmonize with each other in the proper way, a human being can be conceived and then born!

But what happens if they don't? Just what happens with any orchestra.

You can only imagine what would happen if the flutes did not chime in on time or the violins were squeaky, or the conductor didn't time his gestures to the music and whole instrument sections played off key. You would be holding your ears and begging for it to stop! This is what happens when even one or two of these hormones or organs do not work correctly.

A disruption in even one area can lead to many different symptoms of imbalance and suffering for women. There are many symptoms that can result:

- PMS
- Excessive bleeding and cramping
- Clotting
- Bloating

- Breast tenderness
- Weight gain
- Oily skin
- Acne
- Emotional hypersensitivity
- Decreased sexual response or desire
- Hot flashes
- Night sweats
- Insomnia
- Mood swings
- Mental fogginess
- Poor memory
- Migraines or headaches
- Depression
- Fatigue
- Thyroid dysfunction
- Cold hands and feet
- Blood sugar instability
- Gallbladder dysfunction
- Poor muscle tone
- Excess facial hair
- Osteoporosis
- Increased risk of cardiovascular disease

Many unwanted body conditions can occur when our hormonal orchestra is not in tune and playing as it should:

- Endometriosis
- Polycystic ovarian syndrome
- Ovarian cysts

- Cervical dysplasia
- Uterine fibroids
- Infertility
- Irregular periods
- Auto immune disorders
- Copper excess (toxicity)
- Breast cancer
- Endometrial cancer
- Uterine cancer

You may see yourself and some of your own health struggles in these lists of disorders and symptoms. As you start to understand your body more, you can see how and where things can get off track and what to do to help your body heal.

I love the endocrine system. I can feel its ebb and flow in my own body. It is a beautiful rhythm and a wonderful song when all is well. The dissonance we feel in our bodies and the resulting illnesses are often a result of many things going wrong in a distressed body all at once.

Stress can begin at a very early age. Lack of sleep, long nights, chemical solutions, poor diet and seemingly unrelenting life stresses can begin the slow, or in some cases quick, deterioration of the beautiful symphony of our hormones.

CHAPTER 3
The Anatomy of Stress—Your Mighty Adrenal Glands

"HARMONY MAKES SMALL THINGS GROW; LACK OF IT MAKES GREAT THINGS DECAY."

– SALLUST

Introducing your multifunctional and vitally important adrenal glands!

These little glands secrete some of the most important hormones our bodies create. Sitting above the kidneys, they are just about the size of a walnut, but despite their size the adrenals regulate and have a role in the function of almost every organ and tissue in your body. For such small glands, they certainly have a huge part to play in your wellness.

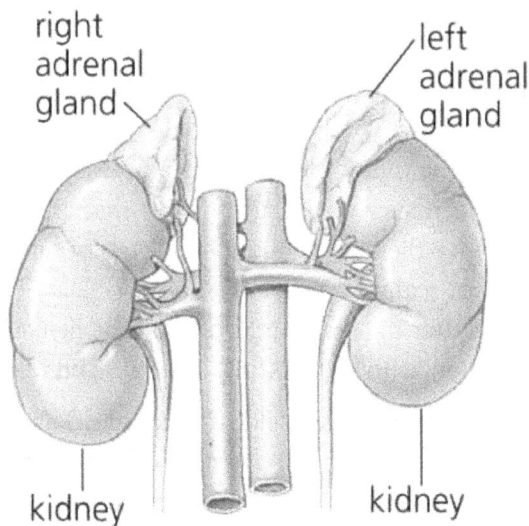

In addition to managing stress, the mighty adrenals manufacture and secrete steroid hormones such as estrogen, testosterone and cortisol. All your female hormones are necessary for health and wellness, and after menopause the adrenals single handedly create the bulk of these hormones all by themselves! If the adrenals have reached a severe level of fatigue by the time you are in your forties, as they have for many women, you are in for a long, hard road ahead.

You will understand their importance when I tell you that the key role of the adrenals is to regulate and help your body manage stress. Stress is a major source of the illness, disease and unhappiness that I see in my patients every day. The adrenals handle stress from all sources. When your body is stressed, the adrenals take over and manage it all the time, whenever it happens, even if that means 24 hours a day, 7 days a week.

I can say with confidence that in our modern society, most of us have lifestyles that are very stressful to maintain. The latest statistics show that we are experiencing more and more stress in increasing amounts. For some, the difficult expectations begin in early childhood as parents are pushing kids to take extremely challenging early paths in school to prepare them for success in secondary school and in college. Some kids are taking the SAT in 4th grade! The world is becoming more and more competitive, and kids learn this lesson very early.

Being a parent myself, I chose the path of sanity for my kids and for me. We stepped off the "well-beaten path" for my oldest and let him choose his own educational journey. He graduated from his high school program first in his class and has been accepted to the college of his choice with an excellent scholarship and 35 hours of college credit. He does not have anxiety and ulcers, nor is he on the multitude of chemical Class II narcotics given to kids today so they can survive in high schools that are often the size of most colleges and give the same amount and levels of school work to kids who may or may not really want this type of work load. He is happy and excited to move on after the six months of gap time he chose to take after high school graduation, with our blessings, to travel and work on his music.

I understand the desire for your child to succeed. I have it too. But you have to ask yourself the question, "At what cost?" Is taking five advanced placement classes at one time the best road for your child? How will that affect their health, their mental state? Is there another path or program that would better suit his or her goals or personality or both? It is okay to color outside of the lines. Not all of us fit into the defined shapes of our society.

Many of the very bright kids are already doing college work early in their high school career. Their work load is incredible, and they feel tremendous stress but continue because this is the path they have been told is imperative for their later success. They must make the grades because grades and the tests are the keys to scholarships and college is very expensive. And so it begins. The "now I have to ..." (fill in the blank) "because if I don't..." (fill in the blank with any horror story of your choosing). The stress—the stress is slowly and surely killing us as a society. The stress that our youngest and brightest and most vulnerable are exposed to at a much too early age.

For many, the chemical "solutions" for stress start very young. I had a young patient who was pushed to the maximum by school and her parents' expectations. Her parents' solution for her was a drug that "helped her focus." It was a Class II narcotic that kids sell in the hallways and on the playgrounds! This set the stage for her to look for other chemical solutions to her stress. She and her parents did not look to the underlying causes of the issue; they just wanted to give her something to "get her through". They could not see another solution. When she went to college and had anxiety, she looked to a drug for the solution. When she could not sleep, a drug. In a few years she will be the thirty-year-old on sleeping pills and anti-depressants, struggling to get through her day exhausted and sick. There is an underlying cause to any health problem, if only we take the time to look and not give up.

Each case is different, of course, but I can tell you this young woman did not have a deficiency of this Class II narcotic in her body. Many kids could benefit from a different school program, and we as parents cannot be afraid to look for other options for our kids. Our kids' futures are in our hands. You cannot fit a square peg in a round hole no matter how hard you push. There are many ways to a destination. Chemical and narcotic solutions do not address underlying causes or fix a wrong school environment, and often create more problems.

In our society today, the stresses a young woman encounters as she enters college or the work force can be quite challenging. Stress can come from many sources: school and work, relationships, financial problems, staying up all night, food allergies and sensitivities, long-term shift work and just trying to do too much. The examples are endless.

In our more primitive incarnations as humans, the "fight or flight" syndrome was over very quickly. We would either run from the threat or stand and fight, and the body's stress response would be completed. Today the stress we are under is often persistent and never ending. It overpowers our thoughts and our day-to-day lives, creating scenarios our ancestors could never have imagined—or our bodies either. The body was not created to handle a 24/7 stress load. When it never has the chance to recover, we are sent down the spiral of ill health very quickly.

The reason the adrenals have their own chapter here is because they are truly the heroes of your story. They are your body's guardian angels, and I want you to understand them because they are the difference between health and vitality, and disease and exhaustion.

I remember how fascinated I was when I first read about the stages of stress and how the body fatigues. Now, I want to help you to see how your body is working for you every minute of every day to keep you healthy. It compensates for our stress, for our terrible diets, for our busy lives.

Hans Selye, MD PhD (1907–1982) was a Hungarian endocrinologist who is often called the Father of Stress. He called his theory of what we call stress the **General Adaptation Syndrome**, or **GAS.**[*]

According to Selye, a stress is an occurrence that could threaten the wellbeing or survival of an organism. Here's what he said about how stress affects the body:

> "Every stress leaves an indelible scar, and the organism pays for its survival after a stressful situation by becoming a little older."

We can only imagine how old we become after so many stresses that start so young for some of us!

Selye describes the stress response by using three stages of fatigue: alarm, resistance and exhaustion.

Stages of GAS

1. Alarm

When a body receives a stress, the "fight or flight" reaction kicks in and the sympathetic or stress response is stimulated. The body musters all its resources, which then set about handling the current stress. This is an

---

[*] selyeinstitute.org

amazingly effective body system when the stress is temporary, but the problems start when it goes on and on.

Hans Selye General Adaptation Syndrome

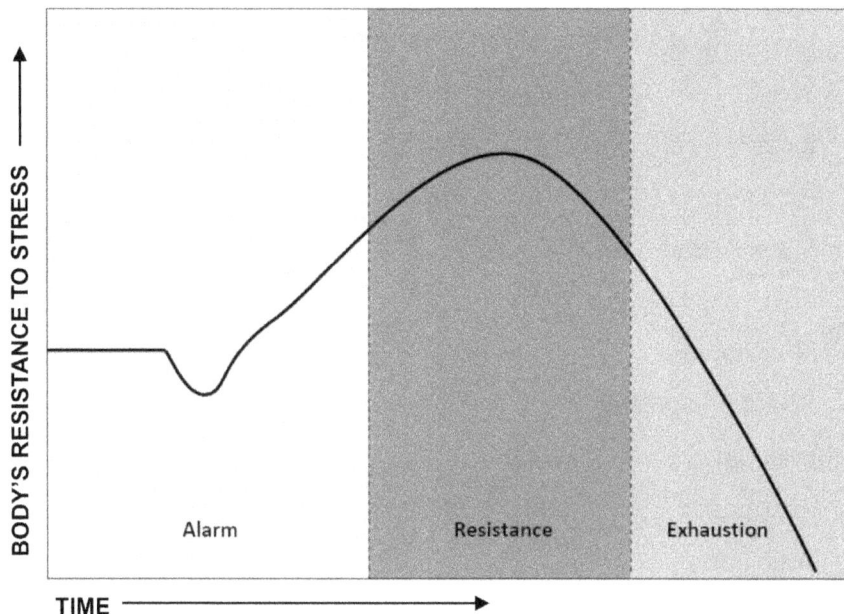

2. Resistance

As the stress continues, the body has a very hard time keeping up this intense response indefinitely. To compensate, it brings in the parasympathetic nervous system—the calming aspect of the body—to attempt to return itself to normal. Meanwhile, it must continue to concentrate on the continuing stress, and never really gets a rest at all. Pretty soon those precious hormones are lessening, and across the board the body is paying the price. More fatigue and exhaustion then begin to set in. Your amazing body is working for you to keep your systems functional despite the ongoing stress, but it grows weary.

3. Exhaustion

As amazing as your body is, it cannot keep up a "code red" situation for days and weeks and months and sometimes years. All the hormones and stress responses that the body has called up are constantly at work to handle the impending threat it perceives. This constant output exhausts the body's resources and organs, and it becomes more susceptible to serious illness and even death. This is when I see most of my patients.

Some of the common symptoms of these levels of adrenal fatigue include:

- Sweet and carbohydrate cravings
- Increased fatigue especially in the afternoon
- Weight gain
- Increased difficulty handling stress
- Anxiousness
- Mood swings
- Memory problems
- Sleep issues
- High blood pressure
- Leaky gut
- Heartburn
- Yeast infections
- PMS
- Infertility
- Decreased libido
- Hypoglycemia
- Impaired immune function
- Inflammation

As we age, and our stress continues, our bodies are striving to keep up. We see the symptoms of this stress showing up daily. Suddenly, our blood pressure is higher when it's always been low, our lipid levels and sugar levels are high when they were always normal in the past. As women age and stress continues, heart disease becomes a very real risk. When we are young we can push through almost anything we encounter. As our stress increases with work and family and children however, those days and years add up. Our resistance is reduced, and illness and disease can set in. We can start to feel very old, very quickly.

I know.

We will talk more about expectations later, but here I want to tell you my own stress story as I think it will help you.

I burned out in graduate school. I had long days and even longer nights. At times, I worked three jobs and still had my standards of all A's to uphold. Because of my perfectionist tendencies I would go and go the extra mile every day to achieve my goals. My body was young and still willing to compensate, but I did my best to wear it out. I ate whatever I could find. Some weeks I measured my stress by how many bags of Doritos I consumed—if it was a really bad week it would be a 3- or even 4-bag Dorito week! I would bake a pan of brownies, eat them all and just collapse on the weekends. The stress was unbelievable—and it took its toll.

I felt very old. I had bags under my eyes. I was exhausted all the time. Unbeknown to myself, I was setting up a foundation for a future of illness. When you push yourself to the limit over and over for years at a time, eat a horrible diet and never sleep, nothing good is going to result. I graduated exhausted, run down and often sick. I was addicted to sugar, and I just thought this was the way it was. I did not even realize I was so tired. It wasn't until much later, after I started my own individualized diet and clinical nutrition health program, that I realized the lights had been out for me for a very long time. When I look back now I can see that I was living way below my potential. I was pushing myself through my days and collapsing at night. I lived on sugar and junk food and coffee. Thankfully, I was never inclined to use chemical crutches, but many of my friends and fellow students did.

It took my adrenals years to recover into a healthy range, so whenever there has been added stress in my life since then—such as childbirth and infants—I make sure my adrenals are well supported. I wonder sometimes how different it would have been if I had known how to eat and how to take care of myself; if I had known to pace myself and to lower my perfectionist standards a bit, and to just eat a balanced diet. If I could have taken some adrenal support—perhaps some whole food adrenal supplements with some B vitamins, especially B5, vitamin C and some herbal adaptogens to help my body deal with the stressors of school and life. If I had even known about the existence of the adrenals, how different would my body have been? How different my health picture?

Staying up all night or into the early morning, not eating regular meals, working the night shift or flying all night on a regular basis as a business person or a flight attendant, eating lots of sugar, continuing a toxic relationship, working in a field you hate, staying in a place that is off your purpose line, not exercising and not addressing chronic stress in your life are all ways you can deplete your adrenal glands and set yourself up for ill health.

Our adrenals are a direct line for all of us to health and wellbeing. They work for us continuously to ensure that we can function and do the things we want to do daily. These vital organs can be depleted and stressed during our early years by our own actions and inactions, our stress loads and our best intentions to succeed. It is so important to know how these glands serve us and how we can help them be at their best, so we can continue to shine through all the stages of our lives as women.

My hope for you is that you learn from my mistakes and ignorance. I would love for the younger ladies that read this to understand this one principle: your body is going to be with you for life. Take care of it. It will take you through your childbearing years, through menopause and beyond. The decisions you make now will determine how easy or how difficult that journey will be.

CHAPTER 4

The Villain of the Piece: Endocrine Disruptors

> "DOCTORS PUT DRUGS OF WHICH
> THEY KNOW LITTLE INTO BODIES OF WHICH
> THEY KNOW LESS FOR DISEASES OF WHICH
> THEY KNOW NOTHING AT ALL."
>
> – VOLTAIRE

NOTE TO READERS: This chapter introduces a topic that is little-known but can be very dangerous to our lives and our health. Reading the facts as I present them can be overwhelming—maybe it's just easier to "give up and hope for the best." Rest assured, this would not be the best decision you ever made. My approach to this problem is simple: You live in the environment you live in. There is no such thing as completely avoiding the toxins I discuss in this chapter. But you can minimize your exposure to them. If your hormone system ever fails from toxic exposure, I have spent twenty years of research working out effective solutions to allow your body to overcome this type of stress.

In the end, your health is only limited by your own willingness to search out and apply effective answers. Giving up? Not the solution at all!

Let's go back to our music analogy. The orchestra is in place and all the instruments are in harmony and blending their voices together in a beautiful symphony. The conductor directs the amazing musicians, and at just the right moment they hit their crescendo. Beautiful sound reverberates in the air—when suddenly a loud squawking is heard from the brass section and a horrible wail begins from the strings section. Violins fly through the air, instruments are dropped, and a black coated band of invaders displace the rightful musicians and begin to play their own version of the piece. Chaos ensues. The conductor is yelling louder and louder, the musicians try in vain to regain their seats and all the while the invaders continue their horrible rendition of the once beautiful song.

This is, in reality, what is happening on a daily basis in your body. Your systems are invaded constantly by toxins that either take the place of or block your body's correct function. Now, instead of correct hormone flow and balanced output, we have what I term endocrine or hormone chaos. Your cycles hurt, you have PMS, you are angry or sad for no apparent reason, your body begins to grow tumors, benign or otherwise, in your uterus or your breasts, you have hot flashes and night sweats, you are exhausted and depressed, your body is no longer yours. It has been hijacked by these foreign substances that now run the show.

These invaders are called endocrine disruptors.

If you are to take full control of your health in our current chemical rich living environment, you must understand these endocrine disruptors, which are mostly manmade chemicals. They are found in pesticides, plastics, plasticizers, metals, additives in food and personal care products, as well as many pharmaceuticals. They include heavy metals such as mercury and lead, dioxin, PCBs, DDT and pesticides, and bisphenol A. These chemicals have long been proven to cause altered reproductive function in both males and females, increase in reproductive cancers in women and men (breast, uterine, ovarian, prostate, testicular) and decreased fertility in both sexes. Neurological and developmental delays have also been seen in children.

As many of these endocrine disruptors mimic estrogen, there has been a substantial increase in the number of women suffering from estrogen dominant conditions. These types of issues include PCOS, ovarian cysts, cervical dysplasia, uterine fibroids, heavy cycles, severe PMS and other female disorders.

We are exposed to these chemicals in our food and our water by inhaling gases and particles in the air and absorption through our skin. One major source of exposure is the transfer of these damaging and extremely harmful chemicals from the pregnant mother to the developing fetus through the placenta, and to the infant and small child through the breast milk. Pregnant women and children are the most vulnerable to these toxins, even though the effects may not be evident until later in life and may even decrease immunity over time.

We all know to some degree that we live in a compromised environment. We read stories about fish or other wildlife dying or being found with genetic mutations or stunted growth in areas of chemical spills. We have all heard of Three Mile Island and similar sites of toxic exposure and the illness and disease that has resulted. But how does this affect you? How does this affect your children? To understand this, you must understand a little more about the structure and the function of endocrine disruptors.

The World Health Organization[*], The Environmental Protection Agency[**] and the National Institute of Environmental Health Sciences (NIEHS)[***] have defined and catalogued the existence of and the damage caused by these endocrine disruptors that are rampant in our environment. I would highly recommend that you link to the NIEHS site and watch the video they have called *Our Chemical Lives.*[****]

What are these horrible, life altering and damaging substances, and where are they found in our day-to-day lives? Many of our everyday personal care products and convenience products contain endocrine disruptors. Some common examples are found in plastic drinking bottles, flame-retardant clothing, toys, cosmetics, pesticides, detergents, birth control pills, conventional HRT (hormone replacement therapy), perfumes, nail polish, soaps, spermicides, adhesives, metal smelting, waste incineration, dry cleaning, dental sealants, food and beverage packaging. This is just a short list of the chemicals found in our clothes, food and the personal care products we may think of as safe for everyday use.

Flame retardants (PBDEs) found in clothing and furniture and other products have been found in increasing quantities in mothers' breast milk. A 2004 report by Ronald Hites, a professor at the School of Public and Environmental Affairs at Indiana University, states that during the past thirty years, PBDE levels in human blood, milk and tissue increased by a factor of 100, essentially doubling every five years.

Hites also conducted a very interesting study that analyzed tree bark to track the spread of these flame-retardant materials in the environmental setting. Tree bark soaks up chemicals from the atmosphere and can be used to help scientists understand how chemical pollution travels in our world. Bark samples were collected from remote locations not associated with the

---

[*] www.who.int/ceh/risks/cehemerging2/en/

[**] www.epa.gov/endocrine-disruption/what-endocrine-disruption

[***] www.niehs.nih.gov/health/topics/agents/endocrine/

[****] www.niehs.nih.gov/health/topics/agents/endocrine/

production or use of the chemicals on five continents. Flame retardants were found in the bark of all the trees sampled, including in a remote region of Tasmania. Flame retardants had managed to travel through the environment and into tree bark in non-civilized areas of our planet.[*]

A recent report by the Environmental Working Group found the average level of the bromine-based flame retardant in American women's breast milk was 75 times higher than the average found in recent European studies. I don't know what you think, but flame retardants should not be in mother's milk! They should not be in salmon or in cow's milk or in the bark of a tree from Tasmania, but they are. The places our children are supposed to be the safest, in our bodies and at our breasts, are where we are inadvertently passing toxins on to our future generations.[**]

How do endocrine disruptors cause damage?

Endocrine disruptors mimic hormones in the body such as estrogen, testosterone, or thyroid hormones. They bind to receptor sites and block the real hormone from binding to its own specific site and then prevent the hormone from completing its action, creating confusion or no action at all. Endocrine disruptors can also block or interfere with the way natural hormones or their receptors are made or controlled.

How Endocrine Disruptors Inhibit Hormone Response

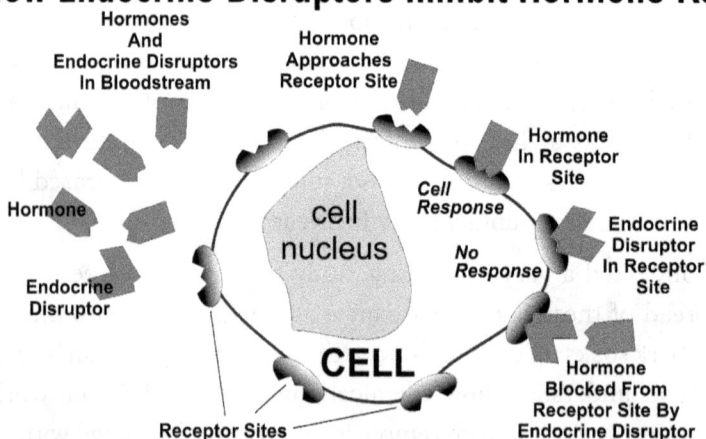

* www.washingtonpost.com/national/health-science/flame-retardants-in-consumer-products-are-linked-to-health-and-cognitive-problems/2013/04/15/f5c7b2aa-8b34-11e2-9838-d62f083ba93f_story.html?noredirect=on&utm_term=.645c99d1c46e

** www.ewg.org/search/site/flame%20retardants%20breast%20milk

Think back to the definition of a hormone we discussed in a previous chapter. Hormones are your body's messenger system. Microscopic amounts of hormone are released directly into the blood stream and exert extremely profound and far-reaching effects on the body. Hormones are measured in nanograms (parts per billion) and pictograms (parts per trillion). Hundreds of different hormones course through our bodies at any given time, at precise times, and in precise measurements, to carry out their duties in the beautiful symphony we've talked about previously.

Endocrine disruptors are the villain of the piece. They are the evil infiltrators come to ruin the magnificent choreography of the body and to disrupt the symphony. They block, damage and destroy these fragile hormones, creating any of the countless health problems you can encounter when your hormones do not work properly.

Worse yet, you are being poisoned by the countless chemicals allowed into our environment. It has been said that over 80,000 man-made chemicals have been introduced into our food and water supply in the last 60 years. Our bodies have not had time to adapt to these chemicals, and most have never been evaluated for health risks in humans. No wonder we as a nation are so sick.

What are the consequences of this flow of toxins into our world and into our bodies? How are they affecting the intelligence and the behavior and the health of our offspring? What is the effect of years of accumulation of these pollutants? No one knows for sure, but we can point to an infertility epidemic, an increase in behavioral and psychological problems, and a very worrisome increase in deaths from all kinds of cancer. Politics and economics combined do not create a climate of quick change—after all, look at how long it took for cigarettes to be "proven" to be bad for your health.

There are many dangers that I and those like me have been warning our patients about for years, and the "establishment" is very slow to accept these things as truth. It is important for all of us to be wise and savvy consumers, to research and to be our own advocates. Trust your intuition. If something seems wrong, it probably is.

When my son was eight years old he would ask me why they showed sugar cereals on TV as healthy and good for children. It is disheartening to tell your child the industry lies and that they advertise things purely for profit in blatant disregard for life and health, but the truth is that they do.

Our Standard American Diet is killing us. If a food has ingredients that you cannot pronounce, and you do not recognize, it is safe to say these ingredients are not good for your body and very well may be endocrine disrupters. Consuming these endocrine disrupters daily is destroying your symphony of health.

End Note:

When I started research on a treatment solution for Endocrine Disruptors back in 2001, the whole subject was considered highly controversial and even pseudo-science. My assertion at the time that most thyroid problems came from or were made worse by endocrine disruptors was considered laughable. Try this: Google "endocrine disruptors and thyroid disease." You'll get more results than you could read in many years, including many papers from the NIH (National Institutes of Health), CDC and every major university.

Obviously, things have changed. We are still a long way from any effective action being taken by industry or government to curb this problem, but awareness and research have expanded exponentially.

Later in this book, I give guidance on avoiding endocrine disruptors and have a section on therapies that help to relieve stress on the body associated with these.

CHAPTER 5
Common Female Health Disorders

This section will give you basic information on common female health complaints and help you better understand how these conditions affect the female body, the medical "causes" (usually unknown), and the medical or conventional treatment options. I am not recommending that you follow or do not follow these common treatment recommendations, because making these recommendations is a job for your medical doctor.

I do, however, want you to see what the conventional medical thought process is on these conditions. Further, I want you to understand that for the most part these conditions have no known medical cause and the treatments consist of drugs or surgery to combat the symptoms or conditions that have already occurred in the body.

I invite you, as you read, to ask yourself the simple question "Why? Why is this happening to the body?"

You see, in other parts of science we learn that for every action there is an equal and opposite reaction. Could this be true in healthcare too? Could it be that there are causes underlying health concerns that come from actions or inactions on our part or of those around us?

I urge you to be curious about how someone could develop a health condition. Are there factors in our environments, in our lifestyles, our stressed cultures, or in our diets that could lead to internal changes that could cause things to go very wrong, where organ systems cease to function as they should, with distressing symptoms and disease processes as the result? This has always been a question I ask. "Why?" If I can still ask "Why?" and not have an answer, then I have not gotten to the bottom of the problem yet. Always ask "Why?" If there is a question, there is an answer. If you do not have the answer yet, keep asking.

Endometriosis

What is it?

Endometriosis is a condition that results when the normal tissue that lines the uterus (endometrium) grows somewhere else in the body. It can grow on the ovaries, the bowel, outside the uterus and sometimes elsewhere in the pelvis or abdomen. As the body goes through its hormone cycle, this sensitive tissue does the same, wreaking havoc on the body. This condition, which affects many women, can cause infertility, heavy periods, pain in the abdomen, low back or pelvis, during intercourse or while urinating or having a bowel movement. These symptoms are often worse during your period.

What causes it?

The cause of this condition is not well understood, and there are several possible explanations. The first of these is called retrograde menstruation. This is when menstrual blood, which contains endometrial cells, flows backwards into the pelvic cavity through the fallopian tubes instead of flowing out of the body. These cells can then stick to the walls of the pelvis or even organs in the area. The tissue thickens and bleeds during each menstrual cycle. As this tissue is in all the wrong places, it causes many problems for many women.

The so-called induction theory supposes that hormones or other immune factors transform the cells of the abdomen or pelvis into endometrial cells. It has also been hypothesized that hormones like estrogen could change the embryonic cells (cells from our earliest fetal development) into endometrial cell implants during puberty. Blood vessels or the lymphatic system could also move these uterine cells to other parts of the body.

After a hysterectomy, C-section or other uterine surgery, endometrial cells may attach to the incision itself or escape into the pelvis. The immune system could also play a role in this condition. The body may be unable to recognize and get rid of this excess tissue that is growing outside the uterus.

I have worked with many women who have this issue. Although it is an extremely upsetting condition and can cause extreme discomfort and pain, often women do not realize they have it until they try to become pregnant.

Treatment

The medical solutions often include surgical procedures to remove the tissue, or hormone treatments such as the birth control pill, progestins and other drugs that block the growth of the endometrial tissue by suppressing the hormones that cause menstruation. In severe cases a total hysterectomy may be the treatment recommended. The problem is that this tricky tissue can often regrow in the body after surgery, causing the need for additional surgical procedures.

Uterine Fibroids

What are they?

Uterine fibroids are a very common benign or non-cancerous tumor in women, and I have seen the instances of fibroids become more frequent in recent years.

Fibroids are made of muscle cells and other cells that grow in and around the uterus. Symptoms can be heavy or painful periods, breakthrough bleeding, feeling "full" in the abdomen, pain during intercourse as well as low back pain and infertility, miscarriage or even early labor. Constipation and frequent urination can also be symptoms of fibroids. I have worked with some women who did not have the common side effects of fibroids like heavy cycles or pain and did not know the growths were there until they felt or actually saw the growths in the area of their lower abdomen. I had a woman come in once who suspected she had a problem and could not understand why she looked three months pregnant. Her uterus was full of fibroids.

What causes them?

The causes of these tumors are unknown. Risk factors seem to be being a woman of reproductive age or having a mother or sister who had fibroids. Black women are more likely to have fibroids, and to have larger fibroids.

Some of the specific causes include:

1. Early menstruation and the use of birth control.

2. Diet. Being overweight, eating a diet high in red meat and low in green vegetables, as well as drinking alcohol, can increase your risk.

3. Vitamin D deficiencies.

4. The heavy flow of menstrual cycles and the resultant blood loss can cause anemia in many women.

What are the consequences?

Fibroids can cause infertility, miscarriage or even sometimes increase the risks of pregnancy complications.

Treatment

The common medical treatments for fibroids can include medications, different types of surgery or even hysterectomy.

Fibroids usually grow slowly and often can shrink after menopause when level of reproductive hormones drop. For some of the surgical procedures, "seedlings"—or extremely small tumors—that may not be detected and removed during surgery and fibroids could eventually regrow.

Interstitial cystitis

What is it?

Interstitial cystitis (IC) can be one of the most frustrating and painful conditions. It is a chronic bladder condition that creates a tremendous amount of discomfort or pain in the bladder and pelvic region. The inflammation and irritation in the bladder can cause scarring and thickening of the bladder. Women have IC more often than men, and the symptoms they experience can include frequent urination, urgency, abdominal pressure, tenderness and sometimes extreme pain in the bladder or pelvis, especially when the bladder fills or empties.

What causes it?

Again, there is no specific known cause for IC, and there are probably many factors that can lead to this disorder. (I have found this to be true of many female health issues—it is not always one thing that causes the problem.)

For IC it is thought that there could be a defect in the lining of the bladder which allows toxic substances to enter and irritate the bladder wall. It is also thought that IC could be an autoimmune condition. Infections, heredity or even allergies could be additional causes of IC. Many people can spot a "trigger" from food or other items that exacerbates or worsens the symptoms of IC.

Some factors that seem to be associated with a higher risk of IC are your sex, having fair skin and red hair, and being thirty or older. IC can also be found in conjunction with other disorders such as irritable bowel syndrome, chronic pain and fibromyalgia.

What are the consequences?

This condition can cause a lower quality of life for many women. Emotional problems linked with pain and interrupted sleep are possible with IC. The irritation can cause the bladder to hold less urine and the frequent urination and pain can interfere with social life and the tasks of everyday living. The pain of IC can cause sexual intimacy to become difficult or impossible.

Treatment

Interstitial cystitis is not an easy condition to treat. Some of the medical treatments involve physical therapy to work with the muscles of the pelvic floor, oral medications and nerve stimulation. A treatment in which the doctor places prescription medication into the bladder through a thin catheter has brought some relief to some women. Surgery is an uncommon treatment for IC, though with severe cases surgical procedures could be used to burn off or surgically remove ulcers present in the bladder.

Polycystic ovarian syndrome (PCOS)

What is it?

Polycystic ovarian syndrome, or PCOS, is a common hormonal disorder that occurs in women of reproductive age. PCOS happens when a woman's ovaries or adrenals produce more testosterone than is normal for her body. The result of this increase can cause cysts (fluid filled sacks) to form on the ovaries. Women with PCOS can have infrequent, irregular or prolonged menstrual periods. Women who are obese are more likely to have PCOS and are at a greater risk of developing diabetes and heart disease.

What causes it?

Again, medicine does not have a clear cause for this condition. The following factors have been seen to be possible causative agents for PCOS.

Insulin, which is produced in the pancreas, helps the body to regulate and use sugar. If the cells of the body become resistant to the action of insulin, (insulin resistance) your blood sugar levels can rise and then as a result more insulin is produced. This excess insulin may increase androgen production, (testosterone) causing difficulty with ovulation.

I have seen in my practice that diet plays an extremely important role in this condition. What raises insulin is sugar, and when the diet is full of sugar insulin levels rise and in many cases the person becomes insulin resistant, causing more rises in insulin and more weight gain and more PCOS symptoms.

A low-grade inflammation of some kind in the body, which can be seen in the production of infection fighting organisms, can stimulate the polycystic ovaries to produce androgens, which leads to other problems linked to the heart and circulatory system. The ovaries themselves can begin to produce abnormally high levels of androgen which create acne and increase growth of body and facial hair. Research has also shown that heredity can play a part in PCOS.

What are the consequences?

Irregular cycles are the most common sign of PCOS. You could have fewer cycles per year or longer time in between cycles, as well as extremely heavy periods. The increased levels of androgens can create excess facial and body hair as well as severe acne and even baldness or thinning hair. Patches of thickened dark brown or black skin can be present as well. If your ovaries contain many cysts, the ovaries themselves may fail to function normally causing more hormone imbalances and symptoms.

PCOS can cause infertility, diabetes and a cluster of conditions including high blood pressure, increased levels of cholesterol and triglycerides called Metabolic Syndrome. Having these conditions greatly increases your risk of cardiovascular disease. A mom who has PCOS also may have increased risk of gestational diabetes or high blood pressure in pregnancy. This can lead to premature birth or miscarriage.

Treatment

Some medical treatments include the birth control pill or progestin therapy. Clomid, Femara or Metformin are other common medications for ovulation or type 2 diabetes control and to lower insulin levels. There are other medications to help control the hair growth.

Stopping smoking, eating healthier foods, and losing weight are all treatments for PCOS. Most overweight women who have PCOS could benefit from losing even 10 pounds, which could help with hormonal balance, in turn helping to regulate the cycle.

Serious health conditions can be very real complications of PCOS. The good news is many of these conditions can be prevented, which we will talk more about later in this book.

Infertility

What is it?

The standard definition of infertility is the inability to become pregnant or conceive after one year or longer of unprotected sex. Older women may be considered infertile after six months of unprotected sex, as fertility declines in direct proportion to age. According to the Mayo Clinic 10-15 percent of couples in the U.S. are infertile.

What causes it?

Infertility can result from many causes. The issue could be with either you or your partner or a combination of factors.

To become pregnant, a woman's body must release an egg from one of the ovaries to be joined with sperm from a male and fertilized. The fertilized egg travels through the fallopian tube and into the uterus, where it must attach to and implant into the uterus.

Anywhere along this pathway problems may arise that can prevent pregnancy from occurring.

Many of the female health conditions we have discussed can be a contributing factor to infertility. I have worked with many women over the years searching for the cause of the often-painful issue of infertility. In my experience, it is very important to have a medical infertility evaluation if you have been unable to become pregnant over the course of one year or more of frequent unprotected sex. There may be simple problems with simple solutions. This evaluation may require a physical examination, including but not limited to a gynecological exam and hormone testing.

Discovering the cause

It is important to know if your hormone levels are healthy and if you are ovulating (releasing eggs from your ovaries) during your cycle. Fertility relies on the body being able to release healthy eggs. The reproductive organs must also be healthy, allowing the egg to pass through the fallopian tubes to join with the sperm. After the egg is fertilized it must be able to first travel to the uterus and then implant in the lining. Tests for female infertility will try to determine if all of these steps are working in a woman's body.

A blood test is usually done to measure hormone levels. A test called a hysterosalpingography evaluates the condition of your uterus and fallopian tubes and looks for blockages or other issues. Contrast dye is injected into your uterus and x-rays are taken to see if the uterine cavity is shaped correctly and to ensure that fluid spills out of the fallopian tubes.

Your eggs can be tested as well, with ovarian reserve testing. This helps to determine the quality and quantity of the eggs available for ovulation. Other tests will check levels of pituitary hormones or ovulatory hormones that contribute to or control the general fertility process. Pelvic ultrasounds look for uterine or fallopian tube disease. Hysteroscopy or laparoscopy are ways to view the internal organs and detect any abnormalities. Genetic testing is also done to determine if there are genetic reasons for infertility.

All the tests above are to determine a women's fertility, but often the man may play a role in infertility and he must be evaluated as well for any abnormality. Male fertility requires that the testicles produce healthy sperm in healthy and viable quantities. The sperm that is ejaculated by the man must reach the woman's vagina and travel into and through the cervix into the uterus. Fertility tests for men will determine if there has been a breakdown in any of these areas.

A male fertility exam will usually include an examination of the genitals and semen analysis, as well as hormone testing for levels of testosterone. In the case of semen samples, more than one sample may be required. Genetic testing, imaging techniques such as ultrasound or even biopsies may be performed to evaluate any abnormalities.

Treatment

Medical treatments for infertility depend on many factors. The cause, if one is found (for many, none is ever found), would lead doctors to creating your treatment protocol. Some causes of infertility cannot be corrected. For instance, your age and the age of your partner could be a factor. Medical treatments for men and women differ.

Sometimes lifestyle changes can be beneficial. Otherwise, certain medications can increase sperm count or surgeries that remove blockages could be performed. In males, sperm retrieval can be used when ejaculation is a problem or when no sperm is present in the ejaculate.

Medically, fertility drugs are the main treatment for female infertility, and there are specialists in these fertility procedures. Treatments can include

1. Stimulating ovulation

2. Intrauterine insemination (IUI) where healthy sperm are placed directly into the uterus at ovulation

3. In vitro fertilization (IVF), which involves the stimulation and retrieval of many mature eggs from the woman, fertilizing them with the man's sperm in the lab and then implanting the embryos into the uterus.

For many women, several different types of treatments may be needed in order to conceive. Some complications of fertility treatments may include multiple pregnancies, painful ovaries, known as ovarian hyperstimulation syndrome (OHSS), in which the ovaries become swollen and painful or even exhibit bleeding and infection, although this is rare.

Fertility is a difficult issue and can be very challenging for the patient and the doctor alike. Sometimes the cause is easily seen and resolved at one end of the fertility spectrum. At the other end, the cause is never found, and a woman may never conceive her own biological child, either naturally or with medical help. I usually see women who do not seem to have a "medical reason" for infertility. Sometimes the cause is very easily spotted and corrected, and pregnancy can result, or it may take many different therapies—alternative or medical or both—to achieve a pregnancy.

Osteoporosis

What is it?

Osteoporosis is a very serious condition characterized by bones that become weak and brittle, so that they can break easily with even mild stresses such as bending over or coughing or even a slight fall. These fractures often occur in the hip, wrist or spine. It's important to understand that bone is living tissue that is constantly being built, broken down and replaced. Osteoporosis occurs when the building of new bone cannot keep up with the removal of old bone.

This condition can affect men and women of all races, but older white and Asian women who are past menopause are at the highest risk. Often there are no symptoms in early stages of bone loss. When the bones become sufficiently weakened there may be back pain, fractured or collapsed vertebra, loss of height, stooped posture or more frequent bone fractures that occur more easily than expected.

What causes it?

When you are younger, your body makes new bone faster than it breaks down the old, so bone mass increases. Peak bone mass is usually reached by most in their early twenties, and during the aging process bone is lost faster than the body can build it back up. The higher your peak bone mass, the less likely you are to develop osteoporosis as you age.

There are many other risk factors for osteoporosis besides race. If you have a number of these factors, it will increase the likelihood that you will develop osteoporosis.

Your sex, (women are more likely to develop osteoporosis than men) your family history and your body frame size may make you more at risk for this condition. If your mother or father or sibling had osteoporosis, or if you have a small body frame, you are often at higher risk of developing osteoporosis.

Hormones play a big role in the development of osteoporosis. The lowering of the female sex hormones, especially estrogen, in women during menopause is one of the strongest factors in developing osteoporosis. Too much thyroid hormone can cause bone loss and can occur with too high a dose of thyroid medication or if you have hyperthyroidism. Overactive parathyroid glands and adrenals can cause osteoporosis as well.

If you have a deficiency in calcium or vitamin D for a very long time, you can have decreased bone density or early bone loss. Eating disorders such as anorexia or surgeries to reduce the size of the stomach or to remove part of the intestine can cause lessened nutrient absorption, including calcium, which can weaken bone.

Long-term use of oral or injected steroids, including prednisone and cortisone, will interfere with the body's ability to rebuild bone. Medications for seizures, heart burn, reflux, and cancer can cause osteoporosis as well. When taking long-term medications, it is important to know these, and all the factors connected to bone health and overall health. Many people do not realize that acid blocking medications taken over a long time can lead to a lack of absorption of vital minerals and to a decalcification of bone, and an osteoporotic condition.

Celiac disease, inflammatory bowel disease, cancer, lupus, multiple myeloma, and rheumatoid arthritis can lead to a higher risk of developing osteoporosis. Sedentary lifestyles, drinking more than two alcoholic drinks per day and tobacco use have been shown to contribute to weak bones.

What are the consequences?

The most serious complications of osteoporosis are bone fractures. Fractures in the hip or spine can result in disability and even death, especially for older people. Vertebrae can weaken so much that they may crumple or collapse, which can cause extreme pain, a hunch back appearance and loss of height.

Treatment

Medical treatments are recommended based on how much bone loss you have experienced. The most widely prescribed drugs for osteoporosis include Fosamax, Actonel, Boniva, Reclast and Atelvia.

These drugs have some extremely serious side effects, including nausea, pain in the abdomen and heartburn. Sometimes fever, headache or muscle aches can be present for up to three days. Using these types of drugs for more than five years can be linked to some rare and very scary problems. In one instance the thighbone cracks and may break completely or another issue could be the onset of osteonecrosis of the jaw where a section of the jaw fails to heal and the jaw bone decays.

Conventional hormone therapy started after menopause, which we discuss in another chapter, is often given to women to help maintain bone density. This treatment comes with its own set of side effects, including an increased risk of blood clots, endometrial cancer, breast cancer and heart disease.

Some women may want to use soy protein, which has a similar action on bone as estrogen does. Soy or any estrogens should be used with caution with anyone who has a family or personal history of breast cancer.

Mood swings, depression and anxiety

As you can probably see from our discussion of female health issues, mood swings, depression, and anxiety are commonly seen when there is hormone imbalance. So many women come into my office having been diagnosed with clinical depression, anxiety and other mood disorders and their only treatment has been a medication for the symptoms. Many of these same women have been told that their health problems are "all in their heads" and instead of causes being found a medication is prescribed.

From my experience, I must unearth the cause of the problem for each individual woman. It may seem funny to think of it this way, but you do not have a deficiency of Prozac or Wellbutrin. You might, however, have a deficiency of magnesium and calcium, of the basic vitamins and minerals that make your body function well. Your ability to digest your food may have become compromised and from this springs a multitude of related problems. You may have been completely physically exhausted for many years, with depleted energy reserves and stressed adrenals and thyroid glands.

When the body is exhausted the first thing it wants to do is sleep and sleep, a sign of physical exhaustion that often mimics other emotional symptoms. How can your body keep pushing itself past its limits? Well it can by using stimulants and drugs and copious amounts of caffeine that mask the true symptoms and push an exhausted body past its breaking point.

You will have a decreased ability to handle stress at this point and your physical body will start to shut down to help you survive. You may not be able to deal with the regular circumstances of life you have been dealing with up to now. You may find yourself becoming anxious for no reason and crying more easily. You may become more irritated or angry than the subject or person deserves. You may also keep it all inside and feel like saying what you feel but you don't. This is when many women reach for help in a prescription because no one has told them there is another option.

When your body is exhausted, so are you. When your energy is depleted, you don't want to exercise or even get out of bed some days. The reason for this is what you need to uncover. Uncover this and you will get your life back.

Here are links to more information on these topics:

www.mayoclinic.org/diseases-conditions/endometriosis/
symptoms-causes/dxc-20236425

www.cdc.gov/reproductivehealth/womensrh/healthconcerns.html

CHAPTER 6
Conditions of the Breasts and Menstruation

Breast lumps

Lumps in your breasts are something to take very seriously. Here are some of the different types of breast lumps that can appear differently in the way they look and feel.

A lump can feel hard or thick, it can have definite borders or be a hard area within the breast tissue. It can be a feeling in an area of your breast that differs from the same area on the opposite breast or even different from the surrounding tissue in the same breast. Any breast changes such as redness, dimpling of the skin or pitting, nipple changes or fluid discharges, pain or tenderness are all signs that should not be ignored. The best thing to do if you have any of these breast changes is to have them fully evaluated by a qualified medical professional.

I have my own experiences with cancer in my family. My mom died of cervical cancer, and I lost my sister to a very virulent form of breast cancer. Her doctors thought her inflammatory breast cancer was mastitis from her recent pregnancy. She went for many months without treatment as a result, even though she complained of breast pain and tenderness or a thickening of the breast tissue all through her pregnancy. It is very important to be in touch with your body and to have any suspicious lump or other abnormality checked immediately. Your chances of surviving a cancer are much better if it is found in an early stage.

I know it sounds strange, but I have known women who were afraid to know what was going on with their bodies and ignored all the signs. They stayed in denial about the issue, refusing to get care until it was too late to do anything about it. Always, knowledge is power. To know what you are dealing with gives you an edge to better understand what your possible treatment options can be.

What causes breast lumps?

In most cases breast lumps are benign or non-cancerous. Some benign causes for breast lumps can be cysts, which are fluid filled sacs in your breast, fibrocystic breasts, lipoma, fibroadenoma or mastitis. These are common causes of benign tumors of the breast but the only way to be sure is to consult with your doctor for a professional and accurate diagnosis.

There are some risk factors that you should be aware of regarding breast cancer. Some of these, such as family history, cannot be changed, but there are lifestyle issues that lead to an increased risk of breast and other cancers that you can control. Smoking increases the risk of breast cancer, especially in premenopausal women. The more alcohol you drink, the greater your risk of developing breast cancer. The most recent studies suggest that even small amounts of alcohol can increase risk.

Being overweight or obese increases the risk of breast cancer and other chronic health issues. It has been found that breast feeding and limiting conventional hormonal therapies can decrease risk of breast cancer. The Mayo Clinic reports that combination hormone therapies after menopause for more than three to five years can increase your risk of breast cancer.

Radiation and environmental pollution exposure increases breast cancer risk. High doses of radiation from diagnostic procedures can also be detrimental to your breast health. You should have these types of tests only when absolutely necessary. Our environmental pollution continues to increase. Exposure to endocrine disruptors in our daily lives has been found to increase risk of cancer.

An unhealthy diet that includes fast foods, sugars, processed foods and a diet deficient in fresh vegetables and fruits has been linked to many other preventable health conditions including diabetes, heart disease and stroke. An unhealthy diet is a very important lifestyle component that can lead to increasing your risk of breast and other cancers.

Treatment

No one wants to ever hear those words, "you have cancer." Believe me, it is life changing. Many of our conventional treatments have progressed, but the most common conventional treatments for breast cancer are surgery, radiation and chemotherapy. The staging and typing of the specific cancer can aid in knowing what types of treatment may work best. For many there is a genetic component.

There has been much in the media about the BRCA1 and BRCA2 genes and what to do if you have them. BRCA1 and BRCA2 are breast cancer genes. Women who have inherited a mutation or a harmful change in either of these genes have a higher risk of developing breast and ovarian cancer. According to the National Cancer Institute, women who have an abnormal BRCA1 or BRCA2 gene have a 60% risk of being diagnosed with breast cancer in their lifetime. If you have a family history of breast cancer, your doctor may recommend this genetic blood test be done for you, or even members of your immediate family.

A famous recent case was that of Angelina Jolie, who decided to have a preventative bilateral mastectomy (surgical removal of both breasts) after her genetic testing showed she had a high risk of developing breast cancer. This and other medical treatments for genetic issues are a very individual decision between a woman and her doctor. Angelina Jolie's surgery and the subsequent discussion has raised the visibility of this type of genetic testing for women. Our technology has advanced so much that it often seems miraculous to me that we can see so much of what is happening with our bodies regarding our own personal genetic code.

It is good to remember, however, that not everything is known. We are learning much more about our genetics and how other variations may play into the known genetics that we can predict now in our bodies. Sometimes the body has other gene variations that select in a way that is protective of the organism even when another gene variant could prove to be detrimental. There is a lot more to learn about our genetic code and how it can help us predict and hopefully prevent serious diseases.

It is extremely important for us as women to keep our bodies healthy but also to get regular female health and breast exams. Finding any health problem early is the best way to prevent future problems. Get to know your body. You are your best friend. Take care of yourself. In the chapter on Breast Health in this book, we will examine some other options for preventative breast care.

Fibrocystic breasts

Fibrocystic breasts are a common condition, suffered by more than half of the female population at some point in their lives. In some women it will cause pain or tenderness and lumpiness in the tissue, especially in the upper outer parts of the breast. These symptoms can be most bothersome just before menstruation.

What causes them?

The exact cause of this condition is not known in medicine. It seems though, that hormones play a big role in fibrocystic breasts, especially estrogen. The fluctuation of hormone levels can cause breast discomfort, lumpy or ropey breast tissue, and many times these feelings of discomfort will lessen or clear completely after the cycle has passed. Nothing in recent literature shows that having fibrocystic breasts increases your risk for breast cancer.

Premenstrual syndrome

Premenstrual syndrome, or PMS, is a very common complaint that can affect as many as three out of four women. This syndrome consists of mood swings, breast swelling or tenderness, exhaustion or fatigue, irritability, cramping, headaches, and cravings. For some women this can be a very mild condition but for others these symptoms, which usually appear predictably in the two weeks before the cycle begins, can be severe and cause several days or even weeks of misery.

What causes it?

The causes of these symptoms are more than likely linked to your hormones. Fluctuations of hormones can cause surges and changes which, when out of balance, can lead to PMS. Neurotransmitters are often affected as well during this time, leading to sleep issues and sometimes anxiety and depression.

I have seen that stress and poor diet can be a very big factor in PMS. Sometimes girls or young women can have a hormonal imbalance at a very young age that is never addressed or even found. Sometimes these girls live with this condition for years and years before they find a solution.

What are the treatments?

Many young girls wind up on birth control pills as a common medical treatment for PMS, which I have seen create different problems down the road for their bodies.

What are the consequences?

For some, PMS symptoms can be mainly physical. Women can experience joint pain, migraines, bloating, constipation or diarrhea as well as acne flare ups and exhaustion. For others, the emotional symptoms of anxiety, crying spells, insomnia, depression, foggy head and tension can be almost unbearable. Some women have a combination of physical and emotional symptoms during this time of the month.

Perimenopause

The prefix *peri* means around. This term describes the time that your body is transitioning into the stage of menopause. You are transitioning towards the time that you will no longer reproduce. This stage of a woman's life usually begins in her forties and can continue for many until her fifties. Some women can enter perimenopause even in their mid-thirties.

The levels of estrogen and progesterone, your main reproductive hormones, start to diminish. Often hormone levels will cycle unevenly, and you may start experiencing menstrual cycles when you do not ovulate. When this occurs, estrogen can be uneven or even dominant compared to progesterone, and hot flashes, insomnia, vaginal dryness or irregular cycles can begin. Your cycles can shorten or lengthen, become lighter or heavier. When you have ceased to cycle for twelve months you are considered to have entered menopause.

What are the symptoms?

There are many symptoms that mark this transition between the reproductive years and menopause. When you experience a persistent change of seven days or more in the length of your menstrual cycle, you are more than likely entering the early stages of perimenopause. If you have sixty days or more between cycles, you may be in late perimenopause.

Hot flashes, insomnia, night sweats, increased mood swings, depression, dry vaginal tissue and increased urinary tract or vaginal infections can be present during perimenopause. As your ovulation becomes more irregular, your fertility decreases as well. It is important, however, to remember that as long as you are having periods, pregnancy is still possible. To avoid pregnancy, use birth control until you have had no periods for twelve months.

You may notice during this time that your libido and sexual desire can change, often because of the physical changes occurring in your body. With decreasing estrogen levels, sex drive can be decreased, bone loss can develop, and your cholesterol levels can change unfavorably. I have seen blood pressure and blood sugar levels also begin to increase during this time. The low-density lipoprotein (LDL)—the "bad cholesterol"—can increase while the high-density lipoprotein (HDL)—the "good cholesterol"—can decrease. Both factors can increase your risk for heart disease.

Going through this time of life is normal and expected. Though it is hard to determine exactly when you enter perimenopause, it is a process and a transition period that leads to the next phase of your life as a woman. It is an important time physically as your body is changing rapidly and special care needs to be given to make sure you handle all the changes this new phase of life can bring to your health and well-being.

Menopause

Menopause is the time of life that marks the end of your reproductive years. If you have gone twelve months without a menstrual cycle, you have entered menopause.

What are the symptoms?

Hot flashes, mood changes, sleep disruption and fatigue can be the markers of this stage of life. Often women will experience a slowed metabolism, which can result in increased weight gain.

Many of the symptoms of perimenopause may seem to flow seamlessly into the phase of menopause. Skipping periods, loss of breast fullness, thinning hair and dry skin can be physical manifestations of decreasing hormones. Night sweats, vaginal dryness, mood changes and other emotional changes can be present as well. Into your late thirties and early forties, your ovaries make less and less estrogen and progesterone. These are the hormones that regulate our menstrual cycles, and as we age our ability to reproduce decreases.

As your hormones decrease, your menstrual cycles may become irregular—either shorter or longer than you are used to—and the quality of the cycle may change. They become heavier or lighter, more frequent or less frequent. At some point your ovaries stop producing eggs, and since you are no longer ovulating your body does not need to menstruate anymore. While menopause is a normal phase for any woman, there are some factors that may cause a woman to enter menopause earlier than she might have normally. Smoking, family history, hysterectomy and some treatments for cancer can cause early menopause.

Studies have been done on menopause in other cultures, and it turns out that we American women experience many side effects and changes during menopause that women in other countries do not. It is clear that we in this country expose ourselves to a tremendous amount of stress. By the time we arrive at menopause our bodies are exhausted, and many of us are experiencing many nutritional deficiencies that lead to other physical ailments. Because of poor diet, sometimes for years, lack of exercise and increased stress, we weigh more than we should, have unhealthier bodies and as a result have a harder time maintaining our health.

What does culture have to do with it?

Apparently, there are many cultural differences between the Eastern and Western perspectives regarding the changes that a woman experiences at this time in her life. The Japanese use the word *konenki*, which translates as "renewal years" and "energy." The word *menopause* comes from French and means "to stop or to pause".

The Study of Women's Health Across the Nation (SWAN) is a multi-site longitudinal study that was created to study the health of women during the middle of life, including physical, biological, psychological and social changes. The study began in 1994 and is now over twenty years long. This study illustrates that there are wide variances of symptoms across cultures and races. African-American women tend to have more hot flashes than Chinese and Japanese women. Rural Mayan women reported no hot flashes. These women look forward to menopause, as in their culture they are considered "wise" and have a place of leadership and power in their community.

Latina women and African-American women tend to enter menopause earlier than white women, and Asian women start menopause a little later. Women who smoke start menopause one to two years earlier than non-smokers. There are many things that make these differences—community and cultural beliefs, genetics, environment and diet may all play a role.

In the SWAN study, it appeared that women, no matter where they lived, faced middle-aged menopausal weight gain. In many areas, however, women did not feel cultural pressure to be thin. Gaining too much weight predisposes us to many health issues and raises the risk of heart disease, strokes and many cancers, but cultural pressures can cause an unrealistic expectation of what is beautiful or accepted in a culture. I work with menopausal women who think they need to be as thin as they were in their twenties, and are extremely upset with themselves if they do not achieve this goal quickly and easily. Your body is different now.

The hormonal changes of menopause might be responsible for making it easier to gain weight around the abdomen, hips and thighs, but hormones do not by themselves make us fat. Lifestyle and genetic factors also play a role in weight gain. As you age, your muscle mass decreases and fat percentages increase. As a result, this decreases the rate at which your body burns its caloric intake. This reason alone makes it more challenging to lose weight. For many women, if you continue to eat the same way you have always eaten and do not increase your physical activity you will more than likely gain weight, gradually or quickly, depending on your diet.

Many women see a gradual increase of weight, perhaps five or so pounds gained per year, which could result in a twenty-pound weight increase over four years. This is a significant amount of weight gain that can create many problems, not the least of which is not fitting into any of your clothes! For someone used to just reducing calories or carbs for a few days and losing five to eight pounds over a few weeks, this can come as quite the unpleasant surprise!

Excess weight increases the risk for Type 2 diabetes, high blood pressure, breathing problems, breast cancer, colon cancer and endometrial cancer, not to mention heart disease and strokes.

Clearly, differences in symptoms during menopause between women of different cultures are not determined completely by biology. If a culture grants women independence or a role that gives them more status after menopause, it stands to reason that this transition may be more positive. If you live in a culture where you become less beautiful or less desirable or likely to "lose your man," as you age, it may be much more of a difficult and stressful transition.

Women in our culture are often seen as sex symbols and are valued for this in movies and in advertising. We are brought up on the idea that a woman is valued for her looks, and as she ages she becomes less valuable. Nothing could be further from the truth, and I am happy that there are so many amazing older female role models in business, politics, entertainment and education to set examples for our younger generation. We women have so much to offer the world in our years after menopause.

In so many ways, life has just begun anew! This time of life should be called meno-start!

Here are links to more information on these topics:

www.mayoclinic.org/diseases-conditions/
endometriosis/symptoms-causes/dxc-20236425

www.cdc.gov/reproductivehealth/womensrh/healthconcerns.html

www.breastcancer.org

CHAPTER 7
The Problems with Conventional Hormone Replacement Therapy and the Pill

Women are rarely fully informed of the potential problems and health hazards that can come with the use of conventional Hormone Replacement Therapy ("HRT") or the birth control pill. It is always amazing to me that we think we can take a precisely running organism like the human body and then insert into it foreign chemicals and unknown substances, which pharmaceutical labs have created specifically and only so that they have a patented product to sell in the marketplace. And then we wonder why the body malfunctions, and in many cases develops cancers and other life-threatening conditions as a result. Based on current studies and concern for your own health and longevity, it is vital that you understand the hormones you are being prescribed, as well as how they affect your health and your life.

We are living longer these days, so we women can possibly spend as much as a third of our lives in menopause! What is menopause?

Menopause as "disease"

In 1966, Robert Wilson, M.D. wrote a book called *Feminine Forever*. He had questionable connections to the drug industry, and therefore had a vested interest in the "treatment" of "a woman's hell" (menopause) by hormone replacement therapy. He told women that, "Menopause is completely preventable," and told them to take estrogen. Synthetic estrogen patented by drug companies became the treatment of choice for those women going through "the change." He called women in menopause "castrates" if they didn't take hormones.

In an NPR report by Joe Neel, he highlights how drug makers preyed on the fears of women. Neel points out that the myths and misconceptions surrounding synthetic hormone use survive to this day.[*]

Following is a direct quote from a 1972 film by the drug maker Ayerst:

---

[*]   www.npr.org/news/specials/hrt/

"The physical alterations that are associated with the menopause may induce emotional changes. When a woman develops hot flashes, sweats, wrinkles on her face, she is quite concerned that she is losing her youth—that she may indeed be losing her husband."

In the film, a woman in a nightgown, sitting in a plaid easy chair in front of a fireplace, says, "My boys are both gone, and my husband is away a great deal with his work. The evenings bother me most. And I think we all give thought to the fact that our husbands might become interested in a younger woman, but I don't dwell on the subject."

What?! Women going through menopause were shown to be old and "washed up" and no longer attractive to their husbands. These lies, and misconceptions of women and the fear of the aging process have long haunted us and destroyed our self-worth and dignity. If women believed these lies—and many women did and still do— this belief was often the path to unneeded surgeries, harmful drugs and often more health problems.

Hysterectomy epidemic

This was also a time when women were having hysterectomies in unprecedented numbers. The solution to many health concerns of women was, and still is, the hysterectomy, and during the two decades between 1965 and 1984 about 12.5 million women in the United States underwent this surgery. The largest number were performed in 1975, when there were 725,000, or 8.6 hysterectomies per 1000 women fifteen years of age or older. Even today, 600,000 hysterectomies are performed each year in the United States.[*]

These numbers are astronomical and disheartening. The solution to the health problems we have is to cut out the female reproductive organs because they aren't needed anymore! One of my patients told me recently—now, in modern 2018—her doctor convinced her that her organs were not necessary and with no cancer or any other major health issue, she is going to have a full hysterectomy.

Women are sometimes scared—scared of cancer, scared of what their organs are doing or might do in the future, scared that no one seems to

---

[*] www.ncbi.nlm.nih.gov/pmc/articles/PMC1350353/pdf/amjph00246-0102.pdf

know what to do. I want to help you understand your body and know that you can do something effective about your body's health problems.

Hormone replacement therapy

The birth of modern hormone replacement therapy came in the sixties. When it was shown that estrogen given alone or unopposed caused the uterine lining to grow and could increase the risk of cancer, the medical establishment suggested adding progesterone to the mix to protect the uterus. They certainly could have used natural forms of progesterone and estrogen, or what is commonly called bioidentical hormones, but of course those couldn't be patented and made into a substance that could be sold. So, as a result, Prempro was born.

Prempro is a combination of a synthetic progesterone called progestin and Premarin, a drug made up of three estrogens called estrone, equilin, and equilenin, which are made from horse urine. Yes, the horse estrogens are natural—but they are natural to female horses, not women! Horse urine is vastly different from human urine. The breakdown in the body of the components of Premarin are biologically stronger and more active. These components have been shown to produce cancer-causing DNA changes. The incidence of breast cancer rises when women take Premarin. Premarin can easily throw a woman into estrogen dominance. An excess of sex hormone-binding globulin can result, which in turn can block thyroid function. Even after studies have shown that giving a woman unopposed estrogen, or estrogen alone, as a therapy can be harmful to her health, it is still being done.

Progestins, or synthetic progesterones, have their own side effects. Most progestins are made by chemically altering the natural progesterone, producing a new chemical that looks like progesterone—but which can be patented. Provera is a common progestin combined with Premarin to make Prempro.

The problems with these drugs are many. Progestin suppresses the natural progesterone in the body, and it disrupts the pathways of the adrenal glands and the sex organs. The steroid hormone pathway is fundamental to energy, and women who take this drug long term can experience chronic fatigue and possibly fibromyalgia, but this type of health issue is not conventionally recognized as a possible side effect of synthetic hormone use.

Other side effects can include depression, anxiety, nervousness, fluid retention and breast tenderness, weight gain, migraines, coronary spasm, angina, menstrual irregularities and more.

The most disturbing of the side effects is coronary spasm. Ninety percent of men who have heart attacks have atherosclerosis or obstruction of coronary arteries, but only 30% of women have this. Most heart attacks in women are caused by coronary artery spasm. Strokes, pulmonary embolism, liver disease, breast cancer and gallbladder disease are other symptoms that can be caused or worsened by synthetic progestins.

Unlike progestins, natural progesterone is a vital hormone needed throughout a woman's life. A woman should normally have more progesterone in her body than estrogen. Estrogen and progesterone function together in the body, and estrogen does not function well without sufficient progesterone.

Hysterectomies are often done because of heavy bleeding, fibroids or endometriosis. Many of these conditions are indications of estrogen dominance and a relative deficiency of natural progesterone. Removing the uterus may stop some of the symptoms, but it does not correct the underlying hormone imbalance. At this point, a woman is often put on unopposed estrogen replacement therapy. The result is usually an increase of other estrogen dominance symptoms like depression, fatigue, muscle aches and pains, gallbladder problems, headaches and more.

Additional treatment might now be antidepressants, gallbladder removal or pain medications, none of which do anything to correct the woman's existing hormone imbalance or to address the root cause of the underlying health issue.

At the outset, though the use of these drug combinations of Premarin and progestin helped to relieve menopausal symptoms, the long-term effects had not been fully studied and were not known. This all changed in 2002 when the Women's Health Initiative (WHI) came out. The study of 16,000 post-menopausal women found that the drugs significantly increased the risk of breast cancer and heart attack. The risk of breast cancer was almost double compared to the placebo group. They stopped the study as women began to experience these terrible effects from the use of the drugs.

Though the results of the WHI have since been called into question, here is a current warning posted on www.drugs.com for the progesterone pill:

WARNING: CARDIOVASCULAR DISORDERS, BREAST CANCER and PROBABLE DEMENTIA FOR ESTROGEN PLUS PROGESTIN THERAPY

Cardiovascular Disorders and Probable Dementia

Estrogens plus progestin therapy should not be used for the prevention of cardiovascular disease or dementia.

The Women's Health Initiative (WHI) Estrogen Plus Progestin sub-study reported increased risks of deep vein thrombosis, pulmonary embolism, stroke and myocardial infarction in postmenopausal women (fifty to seventy-nine years of age) during 5.6 years of treatment with daily oral conjugated estrogens (CE) [0.625 mg] combined with medroxyprogesterone acetate (MPA) [2.5 mg], relative to placebo.

The WHI Memory Study (WHIMS), Estrogen Plus Progestin ancillary study, reported an increased risk of developing probable dementia in postmenopausal women sixty-five years of age or older during 4 years of treatment with daily CE (0.625 mg) combined with MPA (2.5 mg), relative to placebo. It is unknown whether this finding applies to younger postmenopausal women.

Breast Cancer

The WHI Estrogen Plus Progestin sub-study also demonstrated an increased risk of invasive breast cancer.

In the absence of comparable data, these risks should be assumed to be similar for other doses of CE and MPA, and other combinations and dosage forms of estrogens and progestins.

Progestins with estrogens should be prescribed at the lowest effective doses and for the shortest duration consistent with treatment goals and risks for the individual woman.* **

---

* www.drugs.com/pro/progesterone-capsule.html

** www.doiserbia.nb.rs/img/doi/0354-950x/2011/0354-950X1104009S.pdf

The birth control pill

As much as people want babies, they also want to prevent them for myriad reasons.

Birth control has been around for as long as we have been making babies, and its history is quite interesting. In ancient Egypt, women used a combination of dates, honey and acacia, and it seems that when fermented, acacia does have an effect like spermicide.

Around 3000 BC, humans made condoms from fish bladders and animal intestines. Closer to modern times, condoms in 1838 were made from vulcanized rubber.

Birth control has had a very conflicted history. Religion has had opinions regarding reproduction and women's rights that date back into early history.

In March 1873, the United States Congress passed a bill to ban birth control, known as The Comstock Act. Its full name was an "Act of the Suppression of Trade in and Circulation of Obscene Literature and Articles of Immoral Use." This act prohibited advertisements, information or distribution of birth control. It also allowed the post office to confiscate any birth control products it found being sent through the mail. The ban came about because of anti-vice and temperance groups that considered birth control to be obscene and worked to outlaw it.*

Oral contraceptives, otherwise known as the birth control pill, were approved by the FDA on June 23, 1960. The name of the first pill was Enovid, and millions of women began using the pill in the first few years of its introduction. It was almost 100% effective at preventing pregnancy, and gave women more control over their sexuality and family planning. The side effects that developed as a result of this new contraceptive, however, were serious.

Barbara Seaman, women's health advocate, patients' rights advocate, American author and co-founder of the National Women's Health Network in Washington D.C., wrote an important work called The Doctor's Case Against the Pill. It was published in 1969 and presented the facts that high doses of estrogen posed serious and even fatal health risks to women. Doctors were not informing women of these risks, which included heart

---

* family.findlaw.com/reproductive-rights/birth-control-and-the-law-basics.html

attacks, strokes, blood clots, cancer, suicide and depression. This book led to senate hearings in 1970 on the safety of oral contraceptives, and because of these hearings the drug companies were required to include printed warnings on all pill packs about birth control risks and clotting disorders. Today, the pill has a much lower dose of estrogen but still comes with its own set of similar risks, still detailed in that printed warning inside every pill prescription pack as a result of Barbara Seaman's activism.

How does the pill work? The combined pill that most women use today contains synthetic estrogen and progesterone that trick your body into thinking it is pregnant. Mid-cycle, when you would normally ovulate, no egg is released from the ovaries so therefore pregnancy cannot occur. The organs that run the menstrual cycle are shut down and do not function as they normally would. When a woman takes the pill, her natural cycle stops. She has a period because when the artificial hormones stop for a week and she takes the sugar pill, the uterine lining is shed, and often a lighter period results.

Some doctors have even recommended women not having cycles at all. In 2003 there were pills released that enabled a woman to go months without her cycle and, on doctor's recommendation, to have only four menstrual cycles or less a year. Some doctors told patients that no cycles were necessary. Depo Provera is given by an injection that often stops women's cycles for three months at a time. I have seen some extremely negative symptoms and side effects with this injection in some women.

Our bodies ebb and flow with a natural rhythm just as the tides and the moons do. We live in a world that values convenience over balance and in doing so we lose the beauty of our bodies and our cycles. Being female, having a cycle, being fertile are all things to celebrate! Taking time from your life to acknowledge this gift is something that can enrich your life as a woman. The "curse" is really a blessing.

When our cycles are "off" or painful, it is often a sign that our lives or our paths may have veered somewhat from a more balanced existence. Our diets, our exercise levels, our stress may have increased beyond what our bodies can easily handle. It signifies a time for us to regroup, to examine ourselves to see what we can do to bring our lives and our bodies back to a healthier state.

In our modern lives and our modern "must have it all" mentality, we can pay the price for ignoring our natural balance and rhythms. Chemically suppressing our bodies' natural functions can cause many side effects, even death.

One of my favorite books to recommend to patients is *The Pill: Are You Sure It's For You?* One chapter is titled "Dying Not to Get Pregnant". This chapter details the side effects of the pill we aren't told and the ones that could cost us our lives. This same chapter mentions that in 1995 government health ministers went public in Britain about the increased risk of thromboembolism in the third-generation pills. The incidence of pill use went down in Britain at this point, as did the incidence of deep vein thrombosis. Real women die every year from this side effect, as well as from strokes, heart attacks and cancers—deaths that can be related to this form of contraception. We all need to know the risks.

In 2005, the World Health Organization's cancer research group, The International Agency for Research on Cancer, reclassified the pill from a "possible carcinogen" to humans to "carcinogenic" to humans. This places the pill in the Class 1 Carcinogen category, along with asbestos and tobacco. It does appear that the pill is protective against developing ovarian cancer. I am not sure though that, considering the other health concerns, one would choose this path only for this reason. Anything that suppresses ovulation or its frequency, such as full-term pregnancy and breast feeding, are preventive of ovarian cancers as well.

As women are given the pill to "regulate" their cycles, it is important to remember that suppression is not regulation. Taking the pill triples the lifetime risk of breast cancer when taken before the age of 18. It can cause insulin resistance, cervical dysplasia, ovarian cysts, and infertility.

There are many, many other side effects in addition to these. They include Increased risk of thyroid and liver problems, nutritional deficiencies in folic acid, B12, B6, magnesium, manganese, zinc, reduced antioxidant levels especially in the liver and a deficiency of vitamin A. These deficiencies can lead to many more severe health risks. The liver is extremely stressed in attempting to "detoxify" and clear these synthetic substances. This hardworking organ can sometimes be damaged long term with synthetic hormones from the pill and conventional HRT.

Read, educate yourself and learn about other more natural and safe means to protect yourself from unwanted pregnancies. Finding alternative solutions may make the difference between health and ill health. Weigh the risk for yourself, now and for the future. I have worked with many women who after "having their cycles regulated" by the pill for many years were unable to get pregnant for months, if at all, after stopping its use. We spent many months cleaning and rebuilding the body after the damage of long term synthetic hormone use.

Read the warnings in the pill packets carefully and see if you feel that this is the right move for you. There are some links to natural contraception choices at the end of this chapter. We will spend the last half of this book discussing the solutions to hormone imbalance and the endocrine confusion created by the pill and other endocrine disruptors.

Make choices that will help solve your body's health problems instead of making more!

Your body is amazing, and it is capable of amazing healing feats. If you learn to understand your body and how it works, you can also love yourself a little bit more through all the stages of your life and realize you do not have to look young or stay young forever. You are beautiful at every age. I tell patients all day long how beautiful they are. Their faces, with their lines and wrinkles, tell a story, their story. The non-flat tummy and the stretch marks have their own stories to tell as well.

You can age well and be healthy. You can eat right and exercise and find health professionals who will work with you to better understand your body's systems and give you what you need to heal naturally, not synthetically.

Hot flashes, night sweats and menopausal symptoms are real. But there are better solutions than horse urine and cancer-causing synthetic hormones! You are beautiful, and your body is an amazing miracle of systems and organs and hormones. You can be well at any age. Work towards health and wellbeing—not artificial youth. You are a beautiful woman and you are here to share your gifts with the world. There is only one you!

Beneath the Sweater and the Skin

How many years of beauty do I have left?
she asks me.
How many more do you want?
Here. Here is 34. Here is 50.

When you are 80 years old
and your beauty rises in ways
your cells cannot even imagine now
and your wild bones grow luminous and
ripe, having carried the weight
of a passionate life.

When your hair is aflame
with winter
and you have decades of
learning and leaving and loving
sewn into
the corners of your eyes
and your children come home
to find their own history
in your face.

When you know what it feels like to fail
ferociously
and have gained the
capacity
to rise and rise and rise again.

When you can make your tea
on a quiet and ridiculously lonely afternoon
and still have a song in your heart
Queen owl wings beating
beneath the cotton of your sweater.

Because your beauty began there
beneath the sweater and the skin,
remember?

This is when I will take you
into my arms and coo
YOU BRAVE AND GLORIOUS THING
you've come so far.

I see you.
Your beauty is breathtaking.

-Jeannette Encinias

Here are links to more information on these topics:

Natural family planning tools

www.fertilityfriend.com

Natural fertility tracking devices

bit.ly/2oGwd2q

bit.ly/2I4bNso

bit.ly/2I25w0v

Barrier methods of birth control

wb.md/2FQ9xnV

IUD explained

www.emedicinehealth.com/birth_control_intrauterine_devices_iuds/article_em.htm#iud_quick_overview

Fertility tracker

usa.daysy.me

CHAPTER 8
The Best Times of Your Life Should Be ALL the Times of Your Life!

What would it be like if you lived your life to its fullest with the best health possible, making the best decisions and achieving a high level of wellness?

I have imagined how life could and should be if we were taking care of ourselves and had the health and life energy we all want. Of course, there are extenuating circumstances, environmental issues and factors outside our control, but what would your health look like at its best? What would this feel like?

Look at the times of life I discuss in this chapter and compare them to your own experience, and perhaps what it could have been had you known what to do to create it, had you known how to access safe and effective solutions to health problems.

I have often found it helpful to see what an ideal circumstance could be so I can make a more credible goal for the future. I have seen my patients take control of their current health situations right where they are in life and become the ideal picture of what they envisioned their health and their life to be. You can do this at any age and at any time. Envision your life the way you want it to be right now.

The twenties and thirties

This is the time of your life when you should be experiencing all things new. You may be in college or graduate school or pursuing a new job challenge. You may be newly married or beginning your family. At this time of your life your health should be vibrant and your energy abundant as you move and grow and change.

As you move into your twenties and thirties, you should be eating a balanced diet of excellent quality fruits and vegetables and lean, organic, non-processed meat, keeping processed foods, alcohol, caffeine and sugar to a bare minimum. You should be exercising three to four times a week to keep your energy up and your body in shape and sleeping at least seven to eight hours per night.

This is the age when many women choose to start families and may go through pregnancy for the first time. Pregnancy should be a special and amazing part of a woman's life. A new person is coming into the world! A family is being made that will bring joy, and new little people for the family and the world. Pregnancy should be a time of hope and expectations and a time when a woman cares for herself and her future little one. She should be balancing her work and her family life in way that brings joy to herself and others.

Ok, I realize this might sound like a fairy tale! This is how I imagine a balanced healthy life to be. It isn't how it is or was for most of us but think how much better it would be if this was the reality. If you haven't had a family yet, think how wonderful it would be for you to plan YOUR ideal situation and create it! I wish I had. I would have made some changes!

During pregnancy, you and your body have very special needs. Specific supplementation for moms, recommended by an alternative or functional medicine professional, will enable you to keep your energy up and spot any deficiencies before they become a problem. Pregnancy can be very hard on a body, especially one that has had a lot of previous stress. Help from a qualified health practitioner can make the difference between a joyful and healthy pregnancy and one that takes a negative toll on the body, possibly even causing future health concerns.

After your baby arrives, you and your family are overjoyed. This is the time for you to pass along the same healthy habits you practiced during your pregnancy and before to your new child and existing family. Processed foods, fast foods and sugar products are consumed infrequently if at all. Whole foods and natural sugars are used for baking and in drinks. As you live through your twenties and thirties, you start to see the amazing things you can create as a woman, at home and in your career.

If you do not have a family, the twenties and thirties are often a time when you are focused on creating a career and a name for yourself in your area of expertise. Ideally, you are sleeping and eating and balancing work and life in a way that gives you joy and fulfillment. If you are in a stressful work environment, take time to balance yourself, notice the stress and do something effective to address it. This will make you more productive and happier in the long term.

In this balanced scenario, you work hours that allow you to exercise and eat in a healthy manner. If in college or graduate school, you take care of your body and eat and sleep the proper amount so that you can keep your immune system healthy and strong. College, graduate school and new jobs can be very stressful times of life, so good sleep habits, healthy food and specific supplementation to support extreme levels of stress are particularly important.

Taking time to plan out what a balanced life looks like and how you can achieve it can be a life changing decision. Looking back on my life, I realize I just went into situations without planning, knowing I was going to "handle it"—and in many cases I was "handled" by the situation instead! Maybe such is the way of youth, but when taking the next big step in life, understanding and seeing, really seeing, what you want your life to be like can be invaluable. You can learn and benefit from my mistakes.

I wrecked my health in graduate school, and it took me years to recover. I will always have a weakness in my adrenal glands as a result. What a difference it would have made for me if I had understood that while school was certainly going to put me through the wringer, I could come through the stress with my health intact if I ate whole foods, stopped the junk food and sugar, exercised and slept.

Instead, I ate whatever I wanted, with no thought of what it could do to my body. I ate pans of brownies and bags of Doritos and drank extreme amounts of coffee and soft drinks, and had completely unrealistic standards for myself, for my grades, and for life. I did not exercise, and I stressed constantly about my grades and classes and projects. I was sick after final exams every quarter, and lost a relationship that meant a lot to me during this time.

These times can and will shape you, and the results of your choices will be with you perhaps for your entire life. These are the foundational years of your life and your health. Treat yourself well. Know there will be stress. Eat healthy, exercise even if you are stressed—especially if you are stressed. Find ways to handle stress, even if that means taking a quarter off or fewer hours if your health is suffering. Finishing college or graduate school quickly isn't worth it if you lose your health in the process.

Also, at the end of the day, being a perfectionist is the way to early burnout. Being a perfectionist is the recipe for unhappiness and more stress. Take it from a perfectionist! You cannot ever be perfect and if hearing that makes you cringe, you need to take some time right now to realize that trying to control your own life or someone else's within your concept of perfection will not make you happy. In fact, it is a sure route to unhappiness.

What I have learned after many years of being a perfectionist is that living that way hurts. It hurts everyone around you, but mostly you. You may never lose that urge to be perfect, but you can learn to love the imperfections. You can let go and let the world, the grade, the meeting be imperfect sometimes. Yes, you should have high standards, but you have to let yourself fall short of them sometimes without self-recrimination—or for some of us, self-flagellation!

As we see the world through our own lens, we often see others the way we see ourselves. Expecting a loved one to respond to life the way we do and treating them the way we treat ourselves when we make a mistake is not healthy and puts the same heavy burden on them that we put on ourselves. Relationships with friends or others often can't withstand this type of pressure.

You can choose a different way! Choose the way that creates more sanity and more joy. You can find it because it is in you. Make your plan and include a lot of love and patience for yourself!

The forties and fifties

As we head into our forties and fifties, our bodies are changing. We are moving into perimenopause and menopause. Our levels of hormones are lessening. Our bodies are preparing for the rest of our lives and we must prepare as well. Often our metabolism slows and as a result we may need to change our diet and our exercise level. This may be hard because we have been doing things a certain way for quite some time.

I remember my first experience of recognizing that my body had changed somehow when I wasn't looking. I was out playing with my son and running in the back yard. We were playing hide and seek, and I was running as I normally would. I made what I thought was a slick move around a tree to avoid being tagged by my son, and as I darted to one side my foot slipped on the fall leaves, it went one way and my body the other. There was a sound like the breaking of a dry stick, as my little one landed on me saying, "You're 'it' Mommy!" That sound was my ankle breaking almost in two! I held my breath with the pain, trying to stay still so that my son would not be scared.

I was definitely "it." It took me quite a long time to heal, and I was off my feet for almost eight weeks!

I couldn't understand why my body had broken so easily. I did some labs to find out a little more about what was happening with my body and realized my vitamin D levels were extremely low. As a result, I increased my vitamin D and calcium intake to improve my bone health.

I then tested my hormone levels, and to my great surprise I was in perimenopause. What? Wasn't I still twenty-eight? Where did the time go? How did that happen? What was going on?!

In the forties and fifties, ideally, you are still strong but may need to take some special care of your body in some very different ways.

For me, one of these changes was my exercise. In my twenties, I used to work out one to two hours per day, an hour of cardio and an hour of weights. In my forties and fifties, I walked more, and I found the joys of yoga. I do not like to run any more—it hurts my body. I love to hike, and I enjoy weights now, but more in moderation. I do a lot of isometric exercise and exercises that utilize my own body weight. I enjoy Pilates and other regimens that strengthen the core muscles.

I have learned that in this time of my life I must love myself even more than I ever have before. Sometimes this love means changing things like exercise, or parts of my diet that I may have done this way for my whole life, but now needs to be done differently because now my body is different.

At this stage of life, I find it extremely valuable to have my hormones tested and to work towards balance with very specific supplementation and diet choices. There is a tremendous amount of information to be learned by doing functional labs that show hormone output and organ function. It is very important to be screened for nutritional deficiencies that include specific vitamins, minerals and omega-3 oils.

This is the time of life when those little bothersome health issues can become more than a slight inconvenience. Lowered and fluctuating hormones can contribute to severe menstrual problems, the beginning of bone loss and more serious health issues. That extra weight can now become almost impossible to lose, and blood work like cholesterol and blood sugar can start to stray from normal values. Now is the time to take some preventative steps that can save time and your future health.

At this stage of life, you may be raising children still at home, looking forward to grandchildren, working in your chosen career or possibly moving into different fields of interest. At this age, older women may become mentors to younger women. For many, this is a time of life to re-evaluate priorities, a time when you know enough to be able to bring life and work into better balance.

Recently, women have been having children later in life, spending their forties and early fifties rearing children. When this is the case, there is often extreme stress on this age group physically as they rear children, and in many cases work a full-time job or career. Moms who do not work outside the home have just as challenging a job. One of my patients married into a blended family and had three new children plus her own two kids, so her responsibilities jumped tremendously with her marriage and she was exhausted and wiped out. She needed help to be able to maintain her basic family life and schedule. We all choose our paths in life, and they are all challenging in their own ways.

You need to be up to that challenge. You need to be able to get up with energy in the morning, to get all those daily tasks under control at home and at work and still have some energy left to exercise and feed yourself properly. If you are unable to sleep properly, eat regular healthy meals and exercise daily because of work and home tasks, it may be time to re-evaluate your current life choices. I recommend you take another look and determine if these choices are serving you well right now. If not, you have to be brave and make some changes.

I recently worked with a woman who was an amazing artist. She was also a professional working in a field she hated, yet she kept doing it day after day, year after year. She was on three anti-anxiety and anti-depressant medications to help her through her days. For her, everything had become a living hell. I would try to get her to work on her art in her off time and she would always say it was impossible. Finding another job was impossible, moving was impossible. She had created a life where all the possibilities were gone. It had become almost something she had to keep up, so she could keep telling herself it was impossible.

It shouldn't be this way. There should be enjoyment in life. There should be fulfillment.

At this age, you want to be really living and showing your children and others how it is possible to achieve a full and balanced life, full of purpose and love, movement and vitality. You want to be an example to younger women coming up behind you, so they can see that it is possible to achieve health and joy in their lives as well.

The same good fresh diet habits, if started early on, will stand you in good stead now. Avoid processed foods and sugar. Your metabolism has slowed, and that rich, sweet food choice can cause more weight gain than it used to. Sometimes the metabolism can slow so much that it seems impossible to lose weight no matter what you do.

At this time of life, quality sleep is vital. You are headed into hormone transitions and may be experiencing hot flashes and night sweats and other uncomfortable symptoms. Know that changes are coming to your body. Plan to handle them with grace and knowledge. You are becoming the wise woman, and your experience of the world can help a younger generation and those around you to make better and healthier choices for a better life.

Your words, and especially your actions, can be a powerful example to others. You play a vital role in your world and your community. What you do makes a difference, sometimes so profound it is hard to fathom.

Eat well, exercise, get your hormones tested with a functional medicine doctor and be kind and gentle with yourself. You may not have been taught to listen to your body, to be in touch with your body, to understand it, but your body has a lot to say if you will only listen. Listen and trust yourself. Learn what your body is saying and how to interpret its communications.

Our current culture will pop a pill for every ill. In many instances, there are simple drugless solutions for health problems. I have spent my career finding these and putting them to effective use with my patients. This is the age that the "pushing through," the stressing for years and the perfectionist lifestyle can now lead to extremely life-threatening health conditions.

Diabetes, heart disease, osteoporosis and many other health issues can shorten our lives. Many of us have ignored our bodies for years, only to pay the price in our forties and fifties. Ideally, at this age you know your body. You listen to your body. You hear it telling you things are changing, and you make the changes needed to keep yourself energetic and productive. You have a lot to give at this stage of life, and healthy habits can keep you vibrant and forever young in body and in spirit!

The sixties and beyond

I would say with confidence that living in a healthy manner and treating yourself well and with kindness from your twenties through your fifties will determine how you will live in your sixties and beyond. That is not to say that you cannot turn your life and your health around in your sixties and beyond, because you can. It's just easier not to have to come back from diabetes, high blood pressure, heart issues and other serious health concerns that can become lasting parts of your life if you aren't careful.

I have a wonderful patient who turned her whole life around in her sixties and went from three blood pressure medications and being a pre-diabetic to half of a prescription of one blood pressure medication. She lost over twenty-two pounds in less than six months and is happy and energetic and able again to travel and enjoy her retirement. She was, and is, a perfectionist, and this in part helped to create a very stressed mom of four who worked full-time in a very stressful industry and pushed for years beyond what were surely the limits of any normal woman!

Her body broke down in the process while she still clung to the notion that nothing was wrong, and she was fine. She had to because, nothing could be wrong for a woman so many depended on for their very livelihood. In fact, on our first visit together she insisted nothing was wrong and her only problem was a little low back pain! She couldn't easily admit even to herself that something was wrong. This was a pattern she had developed to survive. You can't be sick or have anything wrong because you have so much to do! To admit this for her was like a defeat or a failure. She cried when I asked her how she could be healthy when her doctors could not control her blood pressure with three medications and she was pre-diabetic!

Once she acknowledged she had a problem and it was okay to accept that her body was a little less than perfect, it opened the door to a solution. This beautiful woman had given and given of herself to so many others for so many years and it was time for her to give back to herself. Your sixties and beyond should be filled with joy and as much activity as you want.

You should have the energy and drive to work or travel or garden or paint or walk or start a new hobby or adventure or all of these! For many people, this is the time of their lives when they can complete the legacy they want to leave on this earth. I have friends and patients who are still working in their chosen fields in their sixties and seventies, starting non-profits, teaching, lecturing and traveling for work and pleasure, happily fulfilling their goals and purposes.

This is the time of your life when you have so much to offer. You don't want to be on sixteen medications, fighting for every breath, in doctors' offices for chronic health conditions or having multiple surgeries. You want to be vibrant and alive and feel beautiful and healthy. You want to have energy and do the things that bring your life meaning. These bodies need care, and at every age there are special things we all need to do consistently to be healthy!

We have a lot of life yet to live in our sixties and beyond! Let's live to the fullest, feeling great every day and having true and vibrant health! The first step is wanting to be healthy and the second is finding out how to do it.

Do you see a pattern here? Eating well, exercising for your age and body, working with an alternative professional to help you find *exactly* which nutrients you need for your changing body. These simple things can mean the difference between a happy healthy life and one full of pain and ill health.

CHAPTER 9
The Road Back to Optimum Health

Let's talk about the fat—it's winning!

Okay, ladies, after working with many women for many years with very extreme health concerns, can you guess the most important issue I've found for most women? I can give you a clue. It was not blood values or hormone problems or anxiety, not diabetes and blood pressure or gut health or other potentially life-threatening conditions. You probably guessed it. It was their weight. Working with thousands of people, I have learned a few things about weight and how it relates to health.

Most of us want to fit into our clothes properly. We want to look good in those clothes and not feel as if we are hiding. So, I think now is the time for me to talk about body image. I recently took several months to examine my thoughts on body image and to look more closely at how women's bodies are portrayed in the media. It is appalling!

From a very early age, little girls are taught by television and other media that the desired shape of the female body is skinny—very skinny. I know now that I was a very thin adolescent and teen. That however, didn't matter after I received a comment from a family member when we were out swimming about how I had "sturdy, thick athletic thighs." I must have been thirteen or fourteen. That stuck with me forever and I have always thought of myself as having heavy, fat thighs. I look back on pictures through all the phases of my life and I realize I always thought of myself for many of those years as "less than perfect" or in need of "some kind of weight loss".

That is sad. I would like to go back to my twenty-something self and my thirty-something self and tell them, "You are not fat! Enjoy your body. It is beautiful the way it is." What if that was the message we were given as young girls? What if we had unconditional love and support from our parents and community and ultimately from ourselves. The negative concepts and ideas taught to us as children can stay with us for life.

The women's bodies we see on TV or in the movies are "perfection"—or someone's idea of perfection. That may be what has been deemed ideal, but when we as women internalize that vision and decide we should attempt this image for ourselves, we run into trouble with our own perceptions of our bodies. As a result, we can develop often life-long expectations of ourselves and others' bodies that can be very unhealthy. Whose idea is it anyway that ultra-skinny is beautiful? I applaud the companies who are making ads and doing photo shoots with healthy girls of all shapes and sizes.

I am not advocating obesity. I simply want to point your attention to the fact that the prevailing media image of emaciated girls with glamorous clothes hanging on their ultra-skinny frames is not a healthy model either. For most women and girls that goal is unattainable, not to mention undesirable. This image is completely unrealistic and for most very unhealthy.

Having unhealthy amounts of body fat, on the other hand, can lead to cancer, hormone problems, heart disease, diabetes and many serious health issues. This is plainly seen in the literature. I would like us to teach our kids how to eat to be *healthy*, not skinny. There are many things you can and should do to create a healthy body that is neither too fat nor too thin.

Everyone's body is different and here is where genetics does play a role and sometimes an important one.

You cannot choose to be tall or short. You cannot choose the physical traits your parents passed down to you. You can, however, choose what you eat and how you eat. The problem is that our society has adopted a very unhealthy "common" diet that "everyone" eats. How do you feed your child, for example, whole healthy foods like a container of raw veggies and hummus and chicken breast with salad and fresh fruit, when all the kids around them are eating "lunchables", pizza, potato chips, crackers, and pop tarts?

Food is a social thing. The kid whose parents are trying to teach a healthy way of eating are bucking the eating system. Their kids will be "different", odd or even made fun of in the conventional lunch room setting. The traditional school lunch is for the most part a disaster of fat and sugar and unnecessary carbohydrates. The overload of carbs and sugar and fat in our current American diets from childhood has created a generation of kids who have more allergies, more asthma, more behavior problems and more obesity than ever before.

I have seen patients die from preventable health issues because they couldn't or wouldn't change their diets and life habits. They had raging diabetes and high cholesterol, had sometimes already had heart attacks and surgical stents or a pacemaker, and still would not say "no" to Aunt Jane's famous sweet potatoes, chocolate cake or any number of unhealthy "treats". If you keep telling yourself you "can't eat like this all the time" when everyone else is eating the "good stuff", you've built a mindset that does not allow for change and, as a result, healing.

I have had other patients faced with the same health crisis who do decide to change their diets and their lifestyles and live out a totally different ending to their life story. What is the difference? From my observation, it's the decision. As one of my patients defined it, "The Aha! moment". From the life stories I have observed from my years in practice, some of these people decided to live while others decided to die from lifestyle related ailments. It is hard to watch someone die from their own preventable decision, but it unfortunately occurs every day in ever-increasing numbers. I hope you will be the one who decides to eat to live and not live to eat.

I love carbs and sugar. I think of myself as a forever recovering sugar addict. When I first met my husband, I was very ill. I had gone to an alternative health practitioner who opened my eyes to what was possible in alternative health. The first thing I was told was to stop eating sugar. I told the doctor I didn't eat much sugar. My husband raised an eyebrow. Turns out that, just like any addict, I did not realize I had a problem.

He pulled out all the receipts of my sugar purchases and when I started looking I realized I was eating sugar all day, every day. I even had a jar of Jelly Belly candies on my desk. I had chocolate bars at home. I would stop at the store and buy gum or some chewy candy whenever I felt the urge. I ate cookies and brownies on the weekends. I was addicted, and I did not even realize it. If you love something, you find a way to eat it and I had loved sugar from early on, even as a small child! I had a habit—a sugar habit. It was killing me, and my body was trying to let me know.

I chose to go "cold turkey" off sugar. I had developed a very scary female health issue that I was told was on the verge of cancer. I was told to have surgery, but I did not want to have surgery. I wanted to see if my body could heal itself. Turns out it could, and it did! But that makes the story seem very short and very painless. It was in fact, very hard and extremely challenging to change the eating patterns I had had my whole life. It was hard to make the changes needed in my diet and in my life to create the correct internal environment I needed so that I could heal. It was hard, but it was necessary! I could never have accomplished what I did with my health without making these changes.

I stopped eating sugar in November 1996. It was the holiday season and I was off sugar. I was sick and exhausted and had a good 15 pounds that would not budge (I wonder why!). Going home for the holidays, I didn't get too much support. Folks thought it was weird that I wouldn't eat sugar. What was wrong with sugar? Have a piece of Auntie's pumpkin pie, your mother's cake, a soft drink. I had to say, "Hey, I want to get well, and this is what I need to do. Don't you guys want to help me?" They just looked at me oddly. Their looks seemed to say, "How could something as simple as pumpkin pie be bad for your health? Everyone eats sugar!"

Well, for me it was the years and years of sugar and soft drinks and rich fat- and carb-laden food I had eaten with no regard for health or reason that had landed me here, young and sick. Sugar does a number on your immune system, your endocrine system and almost every other system in your body.

For example, when you consume a mere tablespoon of sugar you can suppress your body's immunity for several hours. Think of what happens when you eat sugar all day as I did.

Immune suppression stops everything. Sugar and carbohydrates, like bread and pasta and crackers and cookies, raise insulin levels and then this extra energy is stored as fat. As all of us can attest, it seems we have unlimited storage areas in our bellies, our thighs, and our bottoms for fat. We have only limited storage for glycogen, that special energy stored in our liver and muscles for between meals. We can store maybe 15 grams of carbs in the liver and other storage locations after a meal. The rest is stored as—you guessed it—fat.

Sugar and Your immune system— Dr. Linus Pauling's forgotten research

Your body has a very efficient system for protecting itself from outside "invaders" such as viruses, bacteria, funguses, etc. The single most important part of this system is the body's ability to identify and destroy any invaders that get inside.

There is a fact that you may not know about your body's immune system: EATING ANY KIND OF SUGAR HAS THE POTENTIAL TO REDUCE YOUR BODY'S DEFENSES BY 75% OR MORE FOR FOUR TO SIX HOURS.

This is not new data. In the 1970s, Dr. Linus Pauling (one of the greatest researchers in the field of microbiology) discovered that vitamin C helps the body to combat the common cold. As part of the same research, Dr. Pauling found that sugar severely slows down this same process.

This is very important to know, as using this information can prevent illness and dramatically assist healing. Because the idea that sugar is "bad" for you is so controversial, I am going to give you a quick, simplified tour through your own immune system, so you can see for yourself what Dr. Pauling discovered.

How Your Body Disposes of Invaders.

Bacteria, viruses, etc. are literally "swallowed" by a special type of cell called a "phagocyte." This is a cell, such as a white blood cell, that engulfs and absorbs waste material, harmful microorganisms, or other foreign bodies in the bloodstream and tissues.

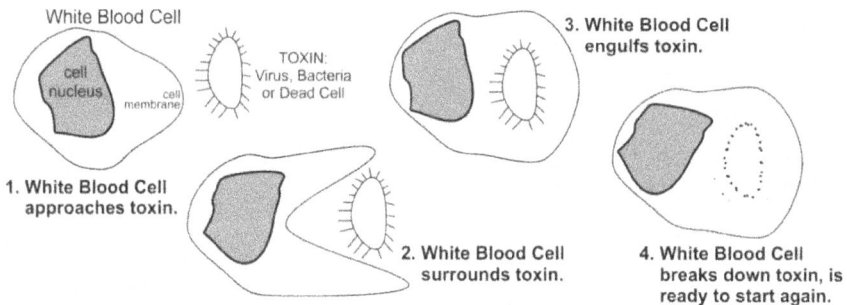

Vitamin C

Dr. Pauling discovered that vitamin C is needed by white blood cells to engulf and absorb viruses and bacteria. In fact, a white blood cell must contain fifty times the concentration of vitamin C as would normally be found in the blood around it. That's how Dr. Pauling came up with the "take vitamin C for a cold" theory. To continue to destroy bacteria and viruses, the white blood cells must accumulate vitamin C all the time to keep up the fifty-times concentration. So vitamin C is being moved through the cell membranes into the white blood cells all over your body all the time. That's why it's important to have plenty of vitamin C available to your body.

Sugar

Glucose (sugar in its simplest form, as found in the blood stream) and vitamin C have a similar chemical structure. So similar, in fact, that when a white blood cell tries to pull in more vitamin C from the blood around it, glucose can get substituted by mistake. If the concentration of glucose in the blood goes beyond a certain concentration, the white blood cell's fifty-times vitamin C concentration can start to drop because of the large amount of glucose it's pulling in as a substitute for vitamin C.

In fact, at a blood sugar level of 120, the white blood cell's ability to absorb and destroy viruses and bacteria is reduced by 75%. This blood sugar level would be easily obtained by any normal person eating some sugar (cake, cookies, candy, soda or even drinking fruit juice). Further, it can take four to six hours for the vitamin C concentration in the white blood cells to reach that optimum fifty-times concentration again.

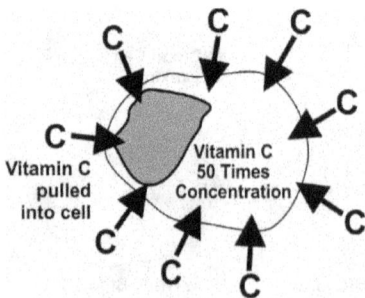

White Blood Cell with 50X Vitamin C, able to destroy toxins in the shortest period of time.

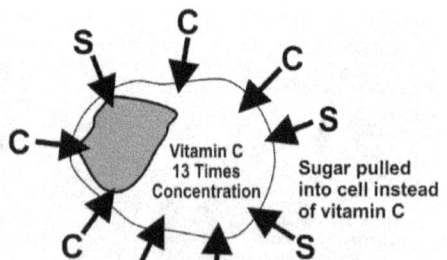

White Blood Cell efficiency is reduced by 75%.

Conclusion

As you can see, it's not a great idea to eat any kind of sugar if you're sick, including the much-recommended orange juice (which may contain vitamin C, but this won't help if the white blood cells can't get past the sugar to use it!). Further, if you were on a program of health improvement of any kind, sugar would be your number-one enemy! White blood cells and other phagocytes remove dead tissue as well as other types of waste associated with injury healing.

The next time you go to the drug store and notice that the cough syrup contains mostly sugar, you can wonder what happened to this valuable research that no one seems to know about!

When someone comes to me and wants to lose weight and has too much fat, what do you think is the cause in most cases? Yes, their diet consists of too much sugar and too many carbs. The amount of sugar we consume in the United States is about 150 pounds per person per year. Scary stuff, but look no further for our obesity and diabetic epidemic. You might try adding up your receipts as I did. I guarantee it will be very enlightening!

You must moderate your carb intake to lose weight in most cases. There are, of course, health issues that would be exceptions, but as a rule you cannot eat 150 pounds of sugar per year (the average American now consumes this amount) and maintain that figure you want to have. Read that last sentence again so that you understand its importance. Many of us want a "special pill" or some type of dispensation from some food god somewhere that will allow us to eat whatever we want and either lose weight or maintain the weight we desire. Unfortunately, it is not going to happen if you do not change your diet. Diet, as many trainers and health professional will tell you, is 85–90% of the problem. You cannot continue to eat chocolate, candy, cookies, pizza, bread, crackers (even gluten free), soft drinks, wine, beer, rum, vodka and many other of these delightful things on a regular basis and expect to lose weight.

As you get older it gets harder. It gets even harder when your adrenal glands are exhausted, and you have hypothyroid concerns. Your female hormones are probably out of balance. As a result, the thyroid is suppressed and the adrenal glands extremely fatigued. Add to that insulin resistance and you are a perfect storm for weight gain. Some women who are swirling in this perfect storm can put on ten to twenty pounds or more in a year.

Now of course we all know someone who is an exception, who can eat carbs all day and never get fat. I am not talking to them, although I would not be confident about their health status overall, especially as they age. If you struggle with your weight, if you have a chubby middle that is hanging over your pants, if you cannot fit into your pants or the pants you want to fit into, look at your diet. Make some changes now. You can do it!

The unrecorded diet is not worth eating!

It is best to record your food intake every day because, like me, you may not realize what you are eating. You may know you don't eat well but you could not say for sure exactly what went into your mouth every day—or you don't want to know! This is a very important recommendation, as it can make the difference between success and failure.

When I work with someone on their weight, I want to see this report, which tells me—and the patient—how many carbs, fats, protein and sugar grams they are consuming daily.

I first realized the value of this in graduate school. In biochemistry class, the teacher had us take samples of our urine for twenty-four hours. We evaluated this urine for fat and carbs and sugar, and oh my! It opened my eyes to the fact that my diet mainly consisted of fat and sugar.

I began to be aware of what I ate, which up to then I had never even thought about. I want you to think about it. I want you to be aware. Ignorance is one thing; willful ignorance is another. At that time in my life, I didn't yet know what do about my diet. If I had known, my life, in terms of my health, would certainly have turned out differently.

Get one of the many online apps or programs for food logging, and just do it for two weeks. Don't change anything—just look at what you are eating. Herein may lie some answers for you, so you must be willing to look. You do not have to "count calories" or points forever but if you want to lose or maintain your weight, use these measurements as a tool. This valuable tracking tool enables you to be mindful and intentional in your eating. It will help you to develop healthy eating habits, and a lifestyle you can live with, to be your best self throughout your life.

You must develop a healthy lifestyle of eating and moving for your future wellness. Imagine a diet that is healthy for you and enables you to have the weight that is healthiest for your body, as well as exercise and movement that you enjoy. If you are ill and need to have a very restricted diet, do this until you are well. Learn what your body needs and must have for wellness. After you have healed and are in a maintenance or wellness phase, you can indulge every now and then in a sweet.

When I was in chiropractic school, I trained with a world-class body builder. I was at my best weight and fitness level during this time. You know what we ate? Egg whites, tuna in water, grilled chicken, lots of salad, vegetables, very small amounts of carbs each day and usually only one or two apples or pears per day—and no sugar at all, ever.

I saw the results in my body. I was hard core with this during this phase in my life. I was about a size four and 120 pounds. I also worked out about two hours a day and spent my life preparing food to eat the "diet", as we called it. I did not ever compete because in my opinion, the competition lifestyle would have been very unhealthy and very obsessive for me. I just loved the workouts and the results. At this time in my life, lean protein and lots of vegetables, a couple servings a day of low-glycemic fruit, no sugar and low-to-no simple carbs was the best diet for my body. I had good body fat and a great BMI—a healthy body I worked hard to create.

Was it easy? No! and no! again. But most of the good things in life are not easy. We had a cheat day once a week and this kept us from going too crazy with cravings, and kept the metabolism moving. Some diets have a "cheat day" worked in and this works for some people—although for some that cheat day becomes a cheat month! I have found overall that it is best to establish a life, including a diet, that you can live with and a lifestyle you can be happy with every day.

I read an article some time ago about realistic workout times and diets related to percentage of body fat for women. When I was younger, I worked out two hours a day, with cardio five to seven times per week and weight training five times a week, as well as a "perfect diet". I had a very low body fat at this time of my life, and I worked for it. Everyone is different, and life can bring some changes too. What was working for me back then may not be the same thing that works now. You must look at your height, your bone structure and your age to determine what weight and body fat percentage is healthy for you. A size two or four is not healthy for many women. We all have different body shapes and sizes. You also must look at how hard you want to exercise and how much time you must give to your workouts.

When I was single and had only myself to care for, I could spend two or more hours per day working out, making my own food and making sure all was well for my week. After I got married and had kids, though, my priorities changed, and my time was divided up differently. As your life changes and new challenges arise it is even more important to eat well. Sometimes your exercise time will be a lot less when job and family life become more prevalent in your daily schedule, but at this point it is essential that you keep it in!

As you consider weight and fat, you may need to examine your relationship with food. Do you eat when you are stressed? Do you eat when you are worried? Do you stop eating when you are stressed or worried? Do you starve yourself or restrict your calories to an extreme? Do you binge eat? Do you overeat? Do you skip meals regularly?

One of my patients had been tracking her diet and realized how much sugar she was eating. As she was observing her own eating habits, she realized she was craving and eating foods emotionally. She has a stressful life, and when she was worrying she would reach for a chocolate or ice cream.

She said this realization was a revelation for her because it allowed her to take a second before she grabbed for something, and just notice what was going on with her and her body. Often, just this bit of time enabled her to realize she was stressed! Sometimes, she said, she realized she was thirsty. Getting herself a cup of water and breathing for a couple of seconds enabled her to become more mindful and realize what was happening, and to make a more intentional choice about her food. This is the key. We must mindfully put ourselves in charge of our decisions.

Food is life giving. There are delicious things out there. I am not saying you can never have any of them. You just need to understand two things.

1. The facts about food—how the body uses it and what it turns into after you eat it.

2. Your own body and its limitations.

Once you know these two things, you will know how to eat and what to do and how to treat your body. Now the choice is simple: to do it or not to do it.

I think of all the rewards of eating healthily, with the resulting energy and great sleep and perhaps longer lifespan, as freedom. You can walk the road of health, choosing to eat those things that feed your body and your health. For your body, it is as if the sun is streaming down, the birds are singing, and you have the day off to wander to a new place and experience life the way you want to. You can wake up feeling good and move your body in a fitness class or go on a walk. You can work and travel and be with your friends and family and bend down to pet your dog without pain.

Compare this to the dark prison of pain and exhaustion, fear and very expensive doctor bills. You cannot travel the way you would like, you are too fat for your favorite clothes, your blood results are betraying you. They show you have borderline diabetes and high cholesterol. You have high blood pressure. You are scared, and the sun becomes the night and the pain doesn't let up in your joints and muscles. You have lost your joy and the sunlight becomes a mockery of the day you spend inside the prison of a very unhealthy body that you don't know how to control.

Choose the light and the sun! Please have an "Aha!" moment today. It is not too late. The hospitals and rehabs are full of those who did not choose wisely on the path of health.

Recently, I sat with a patient who has diabetes. His A1C is 9.5. He eats hot dogs and pastries and desserts and breads all day. He is in his late sixties and has over fifty years of habits to change. I looked him in the eye and I asked him, "What options do you have? You can choose sanity, or you can choose chaos. What you must do is stop eating the things that hurt you and start eating the things that help you."

He said, "I've been eating these things for sixty-seven years!"—as if that made it okay. Eating this way his whole life brought him diabetes, statin drugs and high blood pressure drugs and possibly the cancer he was battling. These combinations of illnesses have made him a prime candidate for a heart attack or stroke.

I am in the ring fighting for people's lives every day. I have seen people die from sudden heart attacks and long, slow and painful, chronic diseases.

With love and concern, I remind you to treat your body well. Feed it what it needs. Ignore the voices that say otherwise!

I asked this patient why he would choose the foods that would bring him ill health and suffering. He said they brought him joy and what was life worth living if he couldn't eat the things he wanted? I asked him to look at that statement for a moment. I asked him if living with light and freedom and without pain might be more worthwhile than daily donuts or hot dogs on white buns.

Was his life more about a piece of food or having quality of life and living with his family and friends in good health? He was quiet for a bit and then he said, "Tell me what to do, Doc. I'll do it." That was it. He decided to live, so we will have another beautiful dad, granddad and husband around to minister to others and to be a vital part of our society for more time to come. This is why I do this work.

Can you, will you, make the decision to live? That's all it is. At the end of the day and after all the justifications and excuses, it's a decision. "Tell me what to do, Doc. I'll do it." Some of the most beautiful words I can hear in my daily practice. This is the first decision on the road back.

Sleep and grow thin

Sleep is a very important part of your health. In recent studies, it has been found that most people have been sleep deprived for years. The time you are sleeping is the time your body uses to heal.

One of the most important things the body needs to lose weight and to heal hormone imbalance is sleep. I have seen the most stressed-out and sick bodies inhabited by people who could not sleep because of health concerns or work issues.

Nurses, flight attendants and other nighttime working people have had their whole sleep/wake cycle disturbed by being up all night, sometimes for many years. A good night's sleep is an invaluable gift. Not being able to sleep signifies an imbalanced body and usually a chronic history of health concerns.

When we sleep we make hormones and neurotransmitters. Our bodies and organs get a chance to regenerate. Sleeping seven or eight hours a day is a must for most people, and some people need more. Some people will say they need less. Everyone's body is different, so you must learn to know yourself and get good and restful sleep every night.

Eat right, eat clean

As a basic rule, you must eat a clean, healthy diet that consists of many different vegetables, which should be a main source of nutrients. By vegetables I mean green lettuces, cucumbers, tomatoes, kale, spinach, chard, mustard greens, collard greens, squash, carrots, celery, beets—the list can be very long. You should have four to six servings a day of vegetables and fruit.

The lowest glycemic-index fruits are cherries, blueberries, blackberries and strawberries. Apples and pears are also healthy choices.

My advice is to eat lean and clean protein. Buy organic meats and chicken, and wild-caught fish.

What you do not eat is as important as what you do eat. Avoid sugar. Stop drinking soft drinks, regular and diet. Start shopping around the edges of the grocery store. Get rid of processed and canned foods, frozen dinners and unhealthy chips and fried snacks. Get the bread out. The wheat of today is very unhealthy—this is not your grandma's wheat. It is often very processed and grown with many pesticides and chemical fertilizers.

Many genetic modifications have been made to a large majority of our foods. No long-term studies have been done on the effects of genetic engineering on your food or on your body. There is pesticide or Roundup Ready grain which has been treated to be able to withstand the spraying of herbicides on the grain itself during its growth and even at its harvest. This increases the levels of pesticides on our foods. More than 90% of all corn and soybean crops grown in the United States are genetically modified.[*]

When I first went into practice, I saw an extremely small number of people with gluten sensitivity. Now I have at least five to ten a month, or more. What has happened? It's hard to say definitively, but for most people it is best to keep wheat intake to a minimum. Wheat and grains are often instigators of inflammation in the body. Fresh vegetables create healing and give our bodies the enzymes and vitamins needed to be well. There is no shortcut for healthy eating.

---

[*] www.time.com/3840073/gmo-food-charts/

Eating healthy takes work, and it can cost more than buying the cheapest food on the shelves. But I can say this with certainty, that you can either pay now with your food and be healthy or you can pay later and be sick—and that bill is a lot more expensive. Good health is vital. When you have your health, you have more options. It's as simple as that. Make the decision now to eat for your life and for your health.

Exercise—let's move!

Your body likes to move. It needs to move. Moving is healthy, it relieves stress and it is important for so many reasons. That being said, everyone's body is in a different condition. What may be healthy and great exercise for one may not be so for another. I have some patients who are tired and stressed and fatigued but they continue over exercising, running twenty miles a day, doing extreme workouts and, in the process, creating a major stress on body systems.

For some it is a foreign idea that exercise could be stressful. Most of us think about exercise as being a good thing, and it is! But if you are exhausted and your exercise takes more energy than it gives you, you may be over-exercising for your specific health situation. As I have mentioned previously, you need to know your body and tailor your exercise accordingly. If you have cardiovascular problems, breathing problems or other major health issues, you must coordinate with your health care provider about the right exercise program for you.

When I see patients in my office, we run very specific tests to determine the body's ability to handle stress. Depending on the outcomes of these tests, we can see what forms of exercise would be best for each person. For most of us, walking is the safest and best exercise we can do for ourselves and our bodies. Just thirty minutes a day can have positive, lasting effects on your health.

Let's discuss the menopause weight gain that just seems to get worse every year even though you haven't changed a thing. It is easier to gain weight as you age, but you do not have to let it win the war! To slow the middle-age spread you must change some things about your lifestyle. It is much easier in menopause to gain fat at the waist and the hips and thighs. You lose muscle mass as you age, and this increased fat makes it much more challenging to maintain a healthy weight.

When you are stressed, or when you do not get enough sleep, you tend to snack more and consume more calories. At holidays and on special occasions or parties it is easy to consume more calories than on a regular day, and all this contributes to the ongoing weight gain. If your metabolism is slow and you have more fat than muscle, these extra calories turn into more fat more easily.

There is no magic formula or magic bullet. You must move! Aerobic activity can help you shed excess pounds and maintain a healthy weight. Strength training is important, as gaining muscle mass aids your body in burning calories faster and more efficiently, which makes it easier to have and maintain a healthy weight. Most adults should exercise vigorously for at least 150 minutes a week, as well as strength training exercises at least twice a week.

If you are trying to lose weight you many need to follow different goals or guidelines for your body. The first essential step—sure to be an unpopular one—is to eat less. For this stage of life, the Mayo Clinic guidelines state that, to *maintain* your current weight—*not* to lose weight—you may need about 200 calories a day less in your fifties than you did in your thirties and forties! This is not good news to most of us.

If you like to enjoy food and love to snack, this can be a difficult pill to swallow. To reduce your calories without decreasing the vital nutrition and vitamins and minerals your body needs, pay attention to what you are eating. Keep track of your diet on an app or program that tracks your calories and fat consumption. Choose vegetables and fruits, unprocessed foods, beans, nuts, fish, and chicken. Replace fried foods and hydrogenated oils with good fats like olive oil, avocado, flax oil and fish oils.

One of the best ways to cut down on needless empty calories is to reduce sugar greatly or remove it from your diet. In the average American diet, almost 300 calories a day come from soft drinks, juice, energy drinks, sweetened tea and coffee and flavored waters. Candies, cakes, cookies, pies, donuts, ice cream and other sweets contribute to our excess caloric intake. Alcohol also adds extra, empty calories to your diet and increases your risk of weight gain.

Remember that weight loss at any age means that you will need to make permanent changes to your diet and lifestyle. Work at finding a lifestyle you can live with and enjoy. A healthier you is a better you. The changes you make now may enable you to enjoy your life and the things and people you love at a higher level of health, and longer than you ever imagined. That, to me, is a lot better than an ice cream cone or a chocolate shake right now. Surround yourself with the support of friends and family and others who wish only success for you!

Stress—weathering the storms of our lives

When faced with the challenges of life, if you do not bend with the storm as a willow, life will pound you and meld you into a form you will not recognize when its work is complete. Stress seems to be our never-ending companion. Stress from our work, our relationships, finances, children and other unknowns that life can unexpectedly throw our way.

The challenge is: how do we deal with it? Stress is a killer. Stress leads to heart attacks and strokes, long term illnesses and mental distress. What we do with our stress will determine the course of our lives.

Exercise is a great stress reliever. For many people, myself included, yoga is an amazing way to learn more about your body, how it moves, what it needs and to help you learn physical strategies to deal with the stress of everyday living. For others, Pilates, Barre, Zumba, CrossFit, interval training and other classes and exercises have made all the difference in how they manage stress.

We as a nation are doing too much, and we are doing too many things at one time. What if, for a moment, you structured your days to reflect the priorities of your health and your body, then those of your family, then those of work—in that order? I hear several gears breaking off for some people, and protests about how impossible that would be. What if you took a real hour for lunch and moved your body for at least thirty minutes every day? If you are the one saying this is impossible, there may be other life decisions that need more examination and thought.

I have a patient whom I have worked with for a long time, who could be described as a very stubborn woman. She was a workaholic. For her the most important thing was work, then making sure the work was done, then making sure the money was enough at work, so her business and her family would do well. The fact that she didn't really spend time with her family seemed to be missing from her calculations. The fact that she didn't exercise at all didn't seem to factor in either, because for her, work was first and everything else came after that.

Things are different for her now, and she worked to make it so. It was not easy, but she never gave up. She eats healthy now and she takes her supplements every day. But her fist is still tightly wedged in the monkey jar of work. She is a hard worker, which is great, but there needs to be a balance between work and life. She has her own work to do in the areas of priorities, as we all do. It begins with the decision to lead a healthy life. You are probably reading this book because you made a similar decision, or you would like to.

I hope eventually this patient will let go of some of her current life priorities and realize that in not letting go she could lose everything. My wish for her is that one day she will plan her business schedule around her workout, around her sleep, around her family instead of the other way around. One day she will decide she needs to hire someone immediately to help her manage her business, so she can take the vacation she hasn't taken in twenty years.

One day she will decide others can do work as well as she can, and she doesn't have to do it all herself. One day she will decide time with her kids when they are young is fleeting and gone in the blink of an eye. One day she will take the time to see to her own spiritual goals and her higher purposes on this tiny spinning globe.

Life is a journey of lessons, and each of us has different ones to learn. Decide to live your life with balance. Live your life the way *you* want to live it. Remember a time when you knew what you wanted to do and how you wanted to do it. Sometimes life takes turns we never saw coming, and we wind up down roads we didn't exactly plan.

At any moment you can decide differently, in your own heart in your own mind. You may not get up the next morning with all your dreams fulfilled, but you can take your next step towards it. My hope for you is that you will decide you are worthy of the self-care and self-love that comes with choosing a healthy life-work balance, and that comes with following your passion and your joy.

One day, you will wake up and plan your business schedule around your exercise schedule, around your sleep schedule, around your family time. If you can't, you will start on the path to making a new life, one that will work around the things that matter most, the things that bring you joy and balance, love and life. These things sharpen you and make you a better person. They puff you up with the helium of life, the laughing gas of existence. They make you whole in the broken places. What better way is there to live?

These are my wishes and my prayers for all of us. A healthy life and a balanced lifestyle emanates from a healthy soul. This will happen when you take the time to know yourself, to listen to your body, to make the decisions that will lead you to the people and things that move you towards a higher level of wellbeing, a higher level of healing.

Whatever your wishes are, whatever you think you cannot do, I am here to remind you that you can. Your decisions can change the course of your own life and they can change the course of all our lives. The ripple in the pool is eternal. Everyone who lives better and whose family lives better helps all of us. If you think you and your problems are an island to yourself, think again.

The strands of life are fragile, and they connect us on many levels. Your decision to make better choices in your life will have a ripple effect on others, sometimes for many generations to come. You are here on this earth for a reason. Find that reason, get healthy and get about the business of living, whatever that means for you. Don't waste any more time. The world needs your light.

The gossamer fibers of life weave through our everyday existence, connecting us to our co-workers, our neighbors, other cultures and other lives. What we say, what we think and what we do makes the difference between light, joy and health, and hatred, pain and death.

We are often bound by the chains of our own minds and our own beliefs. Take stock now and decide to live a life of gratitude filled with dreams for the future, and work hard to make that a reality. The more of us who decide that our lives should be lived with balance, including time for challenging work, time for play, time for family and time for friends, time for proper sleep and clean, organic foods, the easier it will become for all of us. This way, we can change society for the better.

I have found that living from a heart of love and gratitude can make the difference in how I interact with my family and my staff as well as the stranger I meet while I am out. Looking for the positive in life can be hard, but again what are the alternatives? Find a way to choose the path of caring, of loving yourself first, then your family and friends and the world at large.

You are worth it. We are all worth it.

CHAPTER 10
Keeping "The Girls" in the Best of Health

My beautiful sister died from breast cancer. She was not even forty years old when she was diagnosed, and she had an undetected breast cancer while she was pregnant. Who would have thought to look for breast cancer in a pregnant mom? No one would have done a mammogram while she was pregnant. How could someone see a potential breast cancer threat while pregnant? What could be done?

Thermography is a test designed to improve the chances for detecting fast-growing, active tumors between mammogram screenings or when mammography would not be indicated, such as with pregnant women or women under fifty. I often think that if my sister and I had known about this test back then, we could have screened her while she was pregnant and was complaining of burning in her breast and breast discomfort. In her case, her fast moving and extremely active cancer was racing through her body and no one knew. It was misdiagnosed first as a pregnancy reaction and then as mastitis after the baby was born.

If we had done a thermography exam, her invasive cancer would have shown up brighter than a building on fire. We would have seen the extreme heat and we would have been able to get her to treatment much sooner than we did. Maybe it would have made a difference, but I will never know that. In any case, the cancer was not diagnosed until it had already spread and there were no good solutions. Because of this extremely personal experience, thermography holds a special place in my heart.

When I learned about thermography and began to study preventative breast health, I could see the incredible need for this in our current culture and in loving memory of my sister, I started offering preventive breast health programs at my office. I began educating women on how to become aware of their breasts and how to detect early changes in them so that they could reduce their risk of breast cancer and other issues, and in some cases even prevent them.

Cancer is a formidable foe. There are no guarantees with this disease, and some cancers are more virulent and unforgiving than others. Cancer has taken my mom and my sister and has probably touched you in some way as well.

Some cancers are more treatable than others, and some have better outcomes. But all of us have a better chance at good health if we are aware of, and do, the things we know will keep our bodies healthy. I can tell you from personal experience that finding a cancer at a later stage, after it has spread, means limited options and less time to find solutions and healing. If there are ways to know and reduce your risks and take preventative action, most of us would agree this is a logical step to take. If one person can detect early breast changes and prevent this terrible disease it will be worth it. If more of us can take steps to prevent it altogether, that is even better.

Moms, in addition to getting your own thermography, get your daughters a thermography in their late teens and early twenties and establish a baseline of breast temperatures for your bodies. You can then see if there are changes year to year and be able to spot possible problem areas early so that you have time to do something about them. With the breast cancer statistics growing, and until we have a cure for this horrible disease, we must as individual women be personally proactive and do everything we can to decrease our own risk factors and detect any breast abnormalities as early as possible. Thermography can make a very big difference in your life and may enable you to take the actions that could actually save it.

The American College of Clinical Thermology has this to say about thermography:

> *"Canadian researchers recently found that infrared imaging of breast cancers could detect minute temperature variations related to blood flow and demonstrate abnormal patterns associated with the progression of tumors. These images or thermograms of the breast were positive for 83% of breast cancers compared to 61% for clinical breast examination alone and 84% for mammography.*
>
> *"By performing thermography years before conventional mammography, a selected patient population at risk can be monitored more carefully, and then by accurately utilize [sic] mammography or ultrasound as soon as is possible to detect the*

YOUR HORMONES IN HARMONY

actual lesion - (once it has grown large enough and dense enough to be seen on mammographic film), can increase the patient's treatment options and ultimately improve the outcome.

"It is in this role that thermography provides its most practical benefit to the general public and to the medical profession. It is certainly an adjunct to the appropriate usage of mammography and not a competitor. In fact, thermography has the ability to identify patients at the highest risk and actually increase the effective usage of mammographic imaging procedures."

The American Academy of Thermology says that, "Breast thermal imaging is a complementary test to other imaging studies such as Mammography, MRI, or Ultrasound. Extensive literature exists on the use of infrared imaging as a breast risk health assessment. Estrogen dominance, ductal congestion, lymphatic congestion, and angiogenesis are all breast health risk factors that breast thermal imaging can help to identify. Women with dense breasts, fibrocystic disease, small breasts, or who have strong family history for breast disease and want to be more proactive in their breast care often consider breast thermography to help accomplish this need."

I wish my sister could be here to get her thermography exam.

Breast thermography works by observing the heat changes in tissue that can indicate early stages of breast disease. This test offers the opportunity for women to detect changes in breast tissue earlier even than has been possible through breast self-examination, doctor examination or mammography studies alone. It can detect changes in the breast tissue eight to ten years before a lesion will show up on a mammogram.

Thermography can detect subtle metabolic changes that accompany breast pathologies, whether it is cancer, fibrocystic disease, hormone imbalance or other breast abnormalities. Your alternative doctor can then structure a plan and lay out a program for possible further diagnostic procedures or other health changes that can help you prevent illness and increase your overall health.

It is important to note that thermography does not diagnose breast cancer. It is a tool that can be used in conjunction with other established diagnostic tests to give you a chance to be proactive about your breast health.

Thermography is an FDA approved, non-invasive, painless, no touch, state-of-the-art test that does not expose your body to any radiation.

Breast cancer used to be an older woman's disease. Now its prevalence in younger women is growing, and thermography can play a valuable role for women under fifty. The biggest advantage to thermography is helping women to detect breast abnormalities earlier and to aid in establishing risk factors for future breast disease. When thermography is used with other diagnostic procedures, the best and most complete evaluation of breast health can occur.

Once a thermography test is done, the values usually range from one to five, one being the lowest risk and five being the highest. Depending upon the outcome, if needed, I will test the body for stress using muscle reflex testing and other diagnostic labs like hormone tests, or other functional labs that can give additional information needed to address the health issues or nutritional deficiencies found. I then develop a very specific health program for the woman, with follow-up assessments and regular monitoring.

Often, I will refer the patient to a medical doctor for additional diagnostic testing such as a mammogram or an ultra sound, as necessary or indicated. Again, thermography does not diagnose breast cancer. If I see signs of cancer or suspect anything that is not right medically, I will refer to the proper medical provider. Thermography can give us as women a way to work on any issues regarding our breasts on a preventative basis. In my opinion this is the best and most proactive way to approach breast health.

The American College of Clinical Thermology recommend these early detection guidelines: One day there may be a single method for the early detection of breast cancer. Until then, using a combination of methods will increase your chances of detecting cancer in an early stage. These methods include:

- Annual breast thermography screening for women of all ages.
- Mammography, when considered appropriate, for women who are age fifty or older.
- A regular breast examination by a health professional.
- Monthly breast self-examination.

- Personal awareness for changes in the breasts.
- Readiness to discuss quickly any such changes with a doctor.

All these guidelines should be used along with your medical history.

Lymphatic Health

Since there is an extensive network of lymphatic vessels in a woman's breast tissue, it is important to keep this vital system draining. If lymphatic congestion is found, there are several things I recommend for a woman to do. These are all simple and inexpensive.

Rebounding

A very simple solution to getting that lymph moving is to use a rebounder, or a "mini- trampoline". You can bounce while watching television or just listening to music for 10-15 minutes, three to five times a week. Rebounding has been shown to have many other beneficial results, such as helping to firm your arms and legs, hips and stomach. It also helps with balance and is easy on the joints. It is a low impact aerobic exercise that can also strengthen the cardiovascular system.

Dry Brushing

Dry brushing is brushing the skin with a soft body brush in a particular pattern, starting at the feet and then brushing, usually towards the heart. The lymph vessels are usually right below the surface of the skin and it is thought that brushing the skin regularly can help to stimulate the normal lymphatic flow and assist the body in detoxing itself. Since the lymphatics are a big part of the immune system, it makes sense to keep them healthy.

Directions for skin brushing

- Start with a soft brush and move up to a firmer one if it is comfortable. Do not stress your skin or cause irritation from the brush. It is supposed to feel good so it should not hurt.
- The lymph has to come up the legs, defying gravity, until it reaches the heart and chest to drain. To help with lymph flow, brush upwards toward the heart and chest, as this is where the lymphatic system drains.

- Start at the bottom of the feet and brush up the legs in long strokes. You can brush each section eight to ten times. Repeat the process with the arms, starting with the palms of the hands, and sweeping up towards the chest eight to ten times. When you get to the stomach and armpits, continue to brush upward toward the chest. If the brush is soft enough, brush it lightly over the breasts, stroking inward toward the chest. Remember, lightly and gently. No pain.

- You can do the same on the back of your legs and arms. If you have a long handle on your brush, repeat the brushing on your back, working inward toward the middle of the body.

- You should not brush too hard, and there should not be red marks or irritation to the skin. The brushing can stimulate circulation, resulting in a nice energy burst. It is a pleasant way to gently exfoliate your skin and give you a healthy glow!

Phluffing the girls

"Phluffing the girls" was conceived by Cheryl Chapman, R.N. H.N.C., as a result of her personal and clinical experiences.

Cheryl is a breast care advocate dedicated to empowering and educating women about self-breast care. She received her nursing degree in 1965 and earned her certification in therapeutic massage in 1988. Cheryl is an extremely knowledgeable resource for breast health, and it is her passion. I have included her breast health "phluffing routine" here for your use with her blessing.

Remember the breasts have lymphatic tissue in and around them, and it is important to keep the lymph moving. Phluffing is moving the breast tissue gently up and down once a day to stimulate motion and just get that lymph moving again. I started phluffing many years ago when I had painful, very tender breasts. I used this phluffing technique every day at shower time, and in a month or two I had no more breast tenderness at all. I used this technique in conjunction with my Breast Health Essential Oil, and it did wonders for my breast tissue.

My own Breast Health Essential Oil is a blend of lavender, frankincense and myrrh in a carrier oil, usually jojoba. Simply put a few drops on damp hands and apply to damp breasts after a shower. Lean forward and put your hands under your breasts. Cup them under the tissue and "jiggle" them up and down ten times. Then, holding the left breast on the side with the left hand, use the right hand to jiggle the breast gently to the right ten times. Then jiggle the breast gently to the left side ten times as well and repeat the process on the right breast.[*]

This is a simple exercise that encourages lymph movement, puts you in touch with your breasts and can help you spot any breast changes right away. Do it daily, along with the dry brushing, and start some new relaxing routines that stimulate lymph flow and leave you feeling energized and relaxed at the same time.

Breast health essential oil

There are many different blends of breast health oil out there. I make my own blend because I love the calming and relaxing effects of lavender and I want the antimicrobial, antifungal, circulatory and tonic effects of myrrh. Frankincense also supplies anti-inflammatory immune enhancement as well as tonic and disinfectant qualities.

Some essential oils can cause irritation to the skin, especially if applied directly. I use these oils in a blend with a carrier oil such jojoba or almond oil. Essential oils are very strong, and their use will be more beneficial if used in a potency that your body can tolerate well. There are many available tutorials and reference materials on essential oils. If you use them when phluffing the girls, they can be very helpful to your breast health and beneficial to you.

Vitamin D

Having the correct level of vitamin D is one of the easiest things you can do for your breast health as well as your overall health. Keeping your vitamin D levels between 60 and 90 can decrease your risk for developing a number of cancers. Vitamin D is also essential for your immune system, your bone integrity and your nervous system health.

Vitamin D is made when the inactive form of the vitamin is activated by sunlight on your skin. Recent studies have shown that women who have low levels of vitamin D in their blood are at higher risk for developing

---

* Here is the link to Cheryl's Phluffing pamphlet with pictures and additional instructions: www.healingtouchprogram.com/content_assets/docs/current/PhluffingYourGirls1.pdf

breast and other cancers. Many women have no idea what their vitamin D levels are, and as a result, they can be very low. In my practice, I have seen many women who have had extremely low levels of vitamin D, as low as even 8 (the low end of normal is 30) which is extremely dangerous and can cause frequent sickness, fatigue and tiredness, bone and back pain, depression, bone loss, hair loss, and muscle pain. This vitamin may play a major role in controlling the function of breast cells, and may even be able to stop breast cancer cells from growing. Women who have breast cancer often have low vitamin D levels.* **

Ways to get more vitamin D

Exposure to the sunshine without sunscreens for short periods of time—fifteen to twenty minutes, three times a week—can give you a good daily amount of vitamin D.

Although small amounts of sun can be healthy, extreme exposure can increase your risk of skin cancer. You can determine the ultraviolet radiation levels on a daily basis by accessing the UV Index given by the U.S. Environmental Protection Agency and the National Weather Service. This service will tell you the strength of the UV rays on a scale from 1–11, based on your zip code. When the UV levels are moderate to high, it is best to use sunscreen to protect your skin.

Environmental Working Group ranks sunscreens for the safety of their ingredients. Please find a safe sunscreen—you don't want to use one with as much carcinogenic possibility as the sun itself!

Your skin pigmentation, where you live and how many daylight hours you have in your area can make it difficult to get all your vitamin D from sun exposure. You may need to supplement your vitamin D as many of my patients do. What is vital, however, is that you know your vitamin D blood serum level before you start taking a vitamin D supplement. A simple blood test is all that is needed.

While others may suggest a slightly lower amount, I recommend that a woman have a vitamin D level of 60, as it has been found that women with a higher level of vitamin D in their blood have a lower risk of cancer. This is

---

* wb.md/2HJPneZ

** www.sci-news.com/medicine/vitamin-d-cancer-05808.html

an easy risk factor to eliminate. If your doctor is not already testing you for vitamin D, please ask for this simple test.

If your vitamin D levels are very low, it is common for you to be prescribed a 50,000 IU dosage. Too much vitamin D alone is also not healthy and can cause you to have too much calcium in the wrong places in the body, even settling out in your blood vessels and causing possible blockage or disease.

I favor accompanying any high doses of vitamin D with a balance of vitamin K2. These two nutrients are a "dynamic duo" and prevent unhealthy and potentially damaging calcium deposition in the body. For every 5000–10,000 IUs of D3, I would recommend at least 100 mcg of K2. I would like to see the 50,000 IU doses be lower and contain K2 with them. I have seen clinically that low levels of serum vitamin D rise very nicely with dosages of 6000–10,000 IUs per day with K2 added for protection.

Another word of caution. If your levels of vitamin D are very low and you are taking a high dose of vitamin D, get your blood levels tested in a couple of months so that you can see if your supplement is bringing those levels up. It is usually recommended that you take the D3 form of the vitamin rather than the D2 form.

You can also increase your vitamin D intake through the food you eat.

Foods that contain vitamin D are the fatty fishes such as herring and salmon, steelhead trout, mackerel, sardines and oysters. Please remember that you can be exposed to high levels of heavy metals, especially mercury, by eating fish. You can find out what heavy metals are prevalent in fish on the EPA website.

Cod liver oil is a very good source of vitamin D. Fortified milk products such as yogurt and milk are also sources of vitamin D. Some people, however, do not eat dairy products, especially conventional dairy products, and I advise people to avoid dairy for the most part when they are trying to recover their health.

Because of the health issues surrounding it, if you do eat dairy it is important to consume organic dairy products. If you do not eat dairy, make sure you consume other foods that have vitamin D or supplement your diet with a high quality and balanced vitamin D supplement.

Iodine and breast health

Iodine is also extremely important for breast health.

Iodine is a nutrient known as a halogen. (Other halogens are fluorine, chlorine and bromine.) Iodine has been known as a nutrient that prevents the formation of a goiter, which is a swelling of the thyroid gland. It is found concentrated in seaweed in a "level that is 20,000 times that of sea water." *

Iodine was first added to salt by the Morton Salt Company in 1924 at the request of the United States government. The lack of iodine in soil in many parts of the U.S., and the fact that people were not consuming iodine rich foods, contributed to many goiter formations.

Unfortunately, it has been found that just 10% of the iodine in table salt today is bioavailable. Many people are sensitive to salt and are avoiding it because of blood pressure and heart concerns. In our modern world, about 40% of the population is deficient in iodine, due to not eating iodine-rich foods and eating foods grown in iodine-deficient soil.

The common chemicals bromine, fluorine and chlorine can replace the iodine in our cells as they are similar in structure, but they are toxic to our bodies. These toxic elements are present in large quantities in our bread (bromides) and our water supplies (chlorine and fluoride) and toothpastes (fluorides), as well as in medications. Bromine, fluorine and chlorine can reduce iodine absorption and damage your body. If you do not have a filter on your water main at your home or on your shower head, steam from a hot shower or bath causes the chlorine to become a gas, which is literally inhaled into your body, or absorbed into your skin if you are bathing in it.

Iodine is important to the body in many ways. For example, it makes up the thyroid hormones T3 and T4, which control our metabolism. Several years ago, when my sister was battling breast cancer, I learned that iodine has many other functions in our body. A book called *Breast Cancer and Iodine* by David Derry, MD, PhD, opened my eyes to how powerful this nutrient is, and how devastating its deficiency can be. As with vitamin D, iodine is a simple nutrient to supplement and can offer so many positive changes and protections to our health as women.

---

* www.johnappleton.co.nz/media/wysiwyg/docs/WHAT_DO_YOU_KNOW_ABOUT_IODINE.pdf

Iodine is also a very strong antiseptic. Jean Lugol, a French physician, found that iodine will kill bacteria, viruses, fungi and protozoa, and he began using it in hospitals. Dr. Derry says, "Iodine is *sine qua non* (without which it could not be) of fetal development; lack of iodine during pregnancy is the leading cause of intellectual impairment in the world." Iodine plays a huge role as the fetus is developing in utero. Years ago, pregnant women were told to take fluoride tablets, but in the 1960s the FDA banned their use, as fluoride has been found to cause neurological damage in the fetal brain.

In most cities today, we have fluoride in our drinking water. This element competes for iodine and can cause iodine deficiency.

Japanese women, who eat the most iodine in their diets, have the lowest rates of stillbirth and infant mortality in the world. Here are some statistics from the Thyroid Research Journal regarding Japanese statistics linked to the high seaweed intake in their diet.

Japanese health statistics linked to high seaweed intake

"The Japanese are considered one of the world's longest living people, with an extraordinarily low rate of certain types of cancer. A major dietary difference that sets Japan apart from other countries is high iodine intake, with seaweeds the most common source. Here are some astonishing Japanese health statistics, which are possibly related to their high seaweed consumption and iodine intake:

- Japanese average life expectancy (eighty-three years) is five years longer than U.S. average life expectancy (seventy-eight years).

- In 1999 the age-adjusted breast cancer mortality rate was three times higher in the U.S. than in Japan.

- Ten years after arriving in the U.S. (in 1991), the breast cancer incidence rate of immigrants from Japan increased from 20 per 100,000 to 30 per 100,000.

- In 2002, the age-adjusted rate of prostate cancer in Japan was 12.6 per 100,000, while the U.S. rate was almost ten times as high.

- Heart-related deaths in men and women aged thirty-five to seventy-four years are much higher in the U.S. (1,415 per 100,000) than they are in Japan (897 per 100,000).

- In 2004, infant deaths were over twice as high in the U.S. (6.8 per 1,000) as they were in Japan (2.8 per 1,000).[sic]*

In Dr. Derry's book, he writes that iodine can coat incoming allergic proteins to make them nonallergic. He believes that the "origin of autoimmune diseases could relate to inadequate circulating iodine."

Fibrocystic breasts are a very significant problem for many women. In fact, according to some studies, as many as two thirds of American women could be suffering from this breast health issue. Iodine has been found to be an extremely helpful nutrient in the treatment and prevention of fibrocystic breasts.

One of the most fascinating statements regarding breast cancer that Dr. Derry makes in his book is this: "I propose primarily that iodine is the trigger mechanism for apoptosis (natural death of cells) and the main surveillance mechanism for abnormal cells in the body. Iodine triggers the death of cells which are abnormal, and this is the part of a thesis that iodine and thyroid hormone act as a team to provide constant surveillance against abnormal cell development."

What he is saying is that iodine plays a role in not just eliminating cancer cells, but also surveilling and locating abnormal cells in the body and marking them for destruction! This can directly affect not just fibrocystic breast disease but breast cancers as well.

There are many tissues in the body that utilize iodine in addition to the thyroid gland and the breast tissue. While the thyroid gland, the breasts and the ovaries have the most concentrated levels of iodine, other glands that utilize iodine are the salivary glands, the prostate, the bones, gastrointestinal tract, and other tissues and fluids in many other parts of the body. The recommended daily allowance (RDA) in the United States for iodine is 150 micrograms. This amount will provide only the amount necessary to avoid a goiter.

It has been postulated that most of us are iodine deficient. In an iodine loading test, a patient takes 50 mg of iodine/iodide combination and urine is then collected for 24 hours. If a person is not iodine deficient, 90% of the dose would be excreted. Levels below 90% would indicate an iodine-deficient state.

---

* www.thyroidresearchjournal.biomedcentral.com/articles/10.1186/1756-6614-4-14

Iodine is an inexpensive nutrient that can create some very positive changes in the body, but taking large amounts is not something you should attempt without medical supervision. To assess your own iodine needs, please consult a functional medicine doctor or qualified provider to help you understand what your individual needs are.

Symptoms of iodine or thyroid deficiency

- Lethargy
- Brittle hair or nails
- Constant fatigue
- Muscular weakness
- Cold intolerance
- Cold hands and feet
- Unusual weight gain
- Depression
- Hoarseness
- High cholesterol
- Puffy face or skin
- Hair loss
- Infertility
- Menstrual irregularities
- Early menopause
- Dry skin
- Constipation
- Weak heart beat
- Poor memory
- Throat pain
- Difficulty swallowing
- Loss of concentration
- Goiter

- Slow heartbeat
- ADHD
- Developmental delays in children and babies
- Fibrocystic breasts
- Other breast issues or diseases
- Female cancers or diseases
- Thyroid dysfunction

Symptoms of thyroid or iodine excess

- Racing pulse
- Heart palpitations
- Grave's disease
- Iodine-induced hyperthyroidism
- Iodine-induced hypothyroidism
- Thyrotoxicosis
- Iodine poisoning

Too much intake of iodine can create life-threatening changes in the body. Be sure to speak to your doctor about dosage and amounts of iodine and types of foods that you can take into your body that will be safe and help you the most.

Foods high in iodine

- Seaweed
- Cod
- Plain yogurt and other dairy products (preferably organic)
- Meats
- Shrimp
- Egg
- Tuna

Please remember to eat clean and organic versions of any recommended foods to avoid contamination from heavy metals or other endocrine disruptors.

There are many sources of information regarding iodine. Dr. David Brownstein, Dr. Guy Abraham and John Appleton are just a few.[*]

A few words on mammography

Mammograms are the gold standard of diagnosis for breast cancer. The debate rages on regarding who should be screened and who should not, and at what ages. I believe every woman has the right and the obligation to understand the risks connected with regular mammogram screening.

An article from Prevention.com[**] has a very good explanation of the statistics and studies that concern the common screening practices in this country. There are many conflicting studies, and many people fall on either side of the argument. This article does an extremely good job of explaining the false positives and unnecessary treatments that often result from mammogram screening done across the board on every woman, as well as the number of cancers detected and in which age groups. All age groups are not the same, and mammograms before the age of fifty have some limitations. It is safe to say that blanket screening of all women may not be the best way to proceed.

Your cancer risk is your risk and must be evaluated with your medical provider. The Gail Model is a test that can identify your risk of developing breast cancer in the next five years based on several factors, such as family history, age of first menstruation and first pregnancy. Every woman and every body is different. With conflicting information and warring special interests, it is very hard to find the truth. You will continue to see scary statistics regarding getting mammograms and not getting mammograms. If you are a woman who has the genetic propensity to develop breast or other cancers, this is a different case and needs to be addressed accordingly. Please use modern technology and technological advances wisely.

---

[*]   *This is a guide I found helpful regarding iodine supplementation: www.jeffreydachmd. com/wp-content/uploads/2014/03/The-Guide-to-Supplementing-with-Iodine-Stephanie-Burst-ND.pdf*

[**]   www.prevention.com/health/trouble-getting-mammogram-40

Sometimes you can lose sight of the benefits of modern technology by saying, as some patients have said to me, "I will never use medicine, I will not do conventional cancer treatments, I will only use alternative therapies." I have had women come to me with a breast lump they refused to have examined. I have had women come to me with obvious advanced breast cancer who refused medical treatment and any of the technology that exists to help them treat the medical condition they had.

I do not treat any disease process at my office, especially cancer. I help people's bodies be healthier, so their bodies can heal more efficiently. When you have cancer, it has been my experience that you need to know your enemy and meet it with similar aggression. I cannot tell you exactly what this is for you. I do know that doing nothing in the face of cancer is foolhardy, and for many it is a death sentence.

On the other hand, it is always your option to choose your treatment or lack of treatment, and I also respect that. I am also not saying that taking an alternative route to cancer is wrong. I am aware of many very good alternative treatment centers in this country and around the world that test and address specific cancers head on with appropriate treatments, and often very successfully.

What I am saying is use common sense. DO SOMETHING. To use a common example, I have patients who want to pretend they do not have high blood pressure. They do not want to take meds but also do not want to do what it takes alternatively to help their bodies heal. As a person who has chosen the alternative route of healing in my own life, it is not always easy. It is definitely not "take a pill and it will all go away". You often must change your diet, sometimes substantially, and often many aspects of your lifestyle as well. A lot of people are not willing to make these changes. For people who have severe health issues but do not want to change anything about their diet or health, the conventional medical route may be the best route for them, at least in the short term.

My personal view on any medical screening or diagnostic test is that you must be personally informed. You are your own best advocate. You need to do what makes sense to you after reviewing all the data you can find from trusted sources, and discussing this with your doctor or medical practitioner, trusted friends and family. It is your right to choose the tests regarding your breast health you feel best about, after examining all the effects both positive and negative. Educate yourself about the options that exist, and work with a good health practitioner who can guide you.

I personally use thermography once a year to spot metabolic changes in my breast tissue. These changes are often microscopic and are present many years before any cancer ever forms. I act on any changes and get improvement. I get regular "well woman" exams, including breast exams, and have a personal breast health program. I have my hormones and blood tested every six months, and I exercise and make diet changes as needed to keep my body healthy.

I have discussed my cancer risks with my gynecologist and decided what measures I need to take to stay healthy. Today's technology is amazing. If there is a problem that needs further imaging we can do that with mammograms, ultrasounds and now a new technique called Molecular Breast Imaging being done at the Mayo Clinic. This very new technology is combined with the mammogram to detect breast cancer in women with dense breast tissue. Since this test is so new, I am not aware of what side effects there may be, although the test does use a radioactive substance to isolate cancer cells.

My point is that, if needed, imaging and technology exist. If you have a problem, use available imaging technology and read and study about your particular health concern. Find a health team who will do their very best for you and support you in your health choices. Be proactive. Every person and every cancer is different. I believe that all screenings of health need to be individual. If there are risks involved in the screening process, we need to be aware of what they are and be able to weigh those risks against any proposed benefit. Our own risk factors for cancers are extremely individual.

Encouragingly, a project is being done at the University of California's Athena Breast Health Network, called the WISDOM trial. This is a five-year study comparing annual mammogram screening on a risk-based approach for women individually. When we know who is at risk for what cancer, we will hopefully be able to base screening on a risk-based approach and not on blanket recommendations for all women.

Take care of yourself by knowing yourself and your body. Come back to a place of awareness about your body's needs and take stock of where you are right now. Do you need to sleep more, eat less, exercise, lose some weight? Have you had a "well woman" exam or a thermogram for your breasts? Have you established your own breast cancer risks? Do you have a home breast health program?

Start with something simple and do something nice for yourself. Love yourself first. You will be surprised how much good that will bring to you. Take care of your body, take care of your breasts and they will take care of you.

For more information, visit aathermology.org.

CHAPTER 11
Smart Solutions to Endocrine Disruptors in Our Toxic World

Avoiding endocrine disruptors in our lives and in our homes

In our modern world, endocrine disruptors are everywhere. They are in our bath soap, in our shampoo, in our makeup and in the substances we use to clean our homes. It seems that wherever we look there are toxins all around. How do we protect ourselves and our families from the toxic build-up and the damage daily exposure to these poisons can cause us?

One of the biggest ways we are affected by endocrine disruptors is through our delicately balanced hormone system. The beautiful symphony of our hormones is destroyed by these insidious contaminants that block our natural hormones or even mimic hormones, especially estrogen, wreaking havoc in our bodies and on our health. As the name implies, these toxic—and most of the time synthetic—chemicals exist in very high levels in our environment. They enter our bodies through the air we breathe, the water we drink and the soil our plants are grown in. Our bodies were not made to easily process these chemicals, and as a result they cause severe damage to cells and organs. They have been linked to many cancers and other life-threatening diseases.

Some of the common endocrine disruptors we are exposed to on a daily basis are in the very products we rely on for living, such as personal care products, sunscreens, cleansers, bug sprays, makeup, and foods that contain heavy metals such as mercury and lead, pesticides and herbicides. The list is so long that, should you research this topic, you will find the amounts of contaminants in our daily lives are much larger than you would ever think possible. In our modern lives today, it is almost impossible to completely avoid these, but you can significantly reduce your exposure to harmful substances by understanding exactly where these toxins are coming from and taking simple steps to protect yourself and your family.

How have we become such a plastic society? If you Google "plastic waste" you can find images that will horrify you. You'll see mountains of discarded plastics creating a landscape in some areas that rivals pictures of deserted, desolate planets in another solar system.

Bisphenol A (BPA) is a plastic that mimics estrogen (xenoestrogen), and it is found in many everyday products. Think about how much plastic is all around us; in our drawers and cupboards, carrying our food and water, making up computer parts and other machinery, in our drinking water—and the list continues. BPA affects breast health and fertility, and causes reproductive cancers as well as obesity and diabetes. It has been found that fully 90% of us have detectable amounts of BPA in our urine.

One of the best ways to reduce your exposure to this extremely toxic endocrine disrupter is to avoid using canned foods. Unless marked otherwise, almost all cans are coated with BPA—even pet food cans. Aluminum cans that contain soda and beer are lined with BPA. Use glass for food storage and do your best to recycle everything you can.

Choose plastics labeled #1, #2, and #4, which do not contain BPA. You can usually find these numbers on the bottom of the product. Plastics labeled with PC (polycarbonate) or label #7 should be avoided. Make sure you look on the bottom of all the plastic water bottles you are drinking from so you can determine if the bottle you are using is safe.

Avoid microwaving in plastic containers as these chemicals can leech into your food while it is being cooked.

Cheap plastic toys can also be a source of BPA.

Always checking your plastic numbers is a great way to prevent BPA exposure in your home life. Reducing your use of plastics in general makes common sense for the environment. Carrying reusable bags for your groceries and other purchases and using reusable water bottles can decrease your plastic trash. If we all did just a little more towards reducing the plastic waste we create, it would make a big difference to the environment we live in and will leave to a future generation.

Personal care products are a huge source of toxicity and a potential exposure to endocrine disruptors. Your skin is a mass of tiny pores that make up millions of little "mouths" that are ready to take in whatever you place on them. Think about that for a second. Lotions, shampoo, makeup, soap, perfume, anything you put on your skin will be absorbed into your body for better or worse. Read the ingredients list. If these ingredients are going on your skin and they are not food safe, they are all the same headed into your body and organ systems and many of them are toxic to your health!

The same goes for food. When you read a bunch of chemicals on an ingredient list and they are not foods or items that you have ever heard of, remember these ingredients are going into your body. They build up over time and sometimes quite quickly, often causing health problems that are hidden from view because few people think about toxic build-up in their cells from their foods or body care products!

Let's start with something we all need: clean, safe water. A simple thing you can do is to filter your water. This will address fluoride, chlorine, heavy metals, pharmaceutical drug residue and a host of other poisonous, potentially carcinogenic toxins that exist in our tap water today. Water is vital for the body, and healthy, clean water is even more important. A whole house filter on the water main of your house will filter out the chlorine and other toxins. Ordering spring water from a reliable source or using reverse osmosis filters or other filtration systems for drinking water in your home will give you clean and pure water.

An August 2016 study in the Environmental Science & Technology Letters addresses polyfluoroalkyl and perfluoroalky (known as PFASs). These substances, which have been linked with cancer, hormone disruptions and other health problems, are exceeding federally recommended safety levels for six million people in the U.S.. These toxic substances can be found in food wrappings, clothing and in the non-stick, stain resistant and water repellant surfaces that are commonly used in non-stick pots and pans.

The study, led by researchers from the Harvard T.H. Chan School of Public Health and the Harvard John A. Paulson School of Engineering and Applied Sciences, found that drinking water is a main route through which people are exposed to these toxins.

"For many years, chemicals with unknown toxicities, such as PFASs, were allowed to be used and released to the environment, and we now have to face the severe consequences," said lead author

Xindi Hu, a doctoral student in the Department of Environmental Health at Harvard Chan School, Environmental Science and Engineering at SEAS, and Graduate School of Arts and Sciences. "In addition, the actual number of people exposed may be even higher than our study found, because government data or levels of these compounds in drinking water is lacking for almost a third of the U.S. population—about 100 million people." *

The Environmental Working Group (EWG) is a group that analyzes not just drinking water but nearly 50,000 U.S. water utilities in fifty states, and tests for hundreds of toxins. Nearly 19,000 public water systems detected lead at levels which would put a formula-fed baby at risk. The EWG has a Tap Water Database which allows you to enter your zip code to reveal what is really in your tap water.**

I don't know about you, but I always thought it was perfectly safe to just drink water directly from the tap. I do not live in a third world country that has a problem with clean drinking water—or so I thought. We have a Safe Drinking Water Act that was put in place in 1974 to supposedly keep our water safe. The problem is that we have come up with more manmade toxins than this act is currently regulating. Not one chemical has been added to the list of regulated chemicals in drinking water since 1996. That is more than twenty years! According to EWG's water studies, they found more than 160 unregulated contaminants in the tap water in our country. This leads to the conclusion that government agencies are not protecting our drinking water.

According to most health professionals, we are supposed to be drinking eight glasses or more of water per day. Considering that our tap water is a cocktail of chemicals, think of the toxic load we are consuming daily from water that we consider "safe". Over-the-counter meds, prescription antidepressants and other medications, fertilizers and heavy metals—all of these and more have been found in drinking water tests conducted in all fifty states, according to EWG.

As we heard recently in the news, there are cities in our country, such as Flint, Michigan, that have had toxic lead levels in the tap water, poisoning

---

* news.harvard.edu/gazette/story/2016/08/unsafe-levels-of-toxic-chemicals-found-in-drinking-water-of-33-states/

** www.ewg.org/tapwater/#.WgNFY62ZPq0

the people who live there, for quite a long time without this being made public knowledge. Lead is extremely damaging, especially to our babies and young children. Run-off from farms and industry continues to pollute our ground water, creating an environment of toxicity and cancer-causing contaminants that we drink every day. Increased levels of nitrates in drinking water have been found to cause birth defects, bladder cancer and thyroid cancer.

Most water treatment plants cannot filter out medications properly, and it was found in Puget Sound, Washington that 81 different drugs and chemicals were not removed by water treatment methods. Anywhere from 10% to 80% of the drugs in water are not removed during treatment. You could be drinking drug residues from blood-pressure meds, anti-anxiety meds, pain killers, narcotics, birth control pills, hormone pills and more.

Water is a very important part of our lives and our health. Make certain the water you give yourself and your family is clean and pure. It could mean the difference between sickness and health.

The Environmental Working Group's zip code database of tap water enables you to find out what chemicals and contaminants have been detected in your local drinking water. As a result, you can find the primary pollution sources and how to filter these from your home's water supply. It only takes a few seconds, but it will open your eyes to what you are drinking from your tap. You can find the information on the group's website.[*]

I entered the zip code for my county here in the Atlanta area, and these were the chemicals found at levels above safe for human consumption:

CHEMICAL	RISK
Bromodichloromethane	Cancer
Chlorate	Thyroid harm
Chloroform	Cancer
Chromium (hexavalent)	Cancer
Dibromochloromethane	Cancer
Dichloroacetic acid	Cancer
Total trihalomethanes (TTHMs)	Cancer

[*] www.ewg.org/tapwater/#.WgNFY62ZPq0

Chemical	Risk
Trichloroacetic acid	Cancer
Radiological contaminants	Cancer

Additional contaminants included haloacetic acids (HAA5), strontium, vanadium, fluoride, nitrates and nitrites.

As I read the lists of chemicals in my home tap water, I was appalled and scared for myself and my family, but also for my community. According to www.cancer.gov, the number of new cancer cases will rise to 22 million within the next two decades. How hard is it for any logical person to wonder if these huge amounts of cancer-causing substances we consume daily in our very food and water could be a contributing factor in the causes of many cancers?

These chemicals and contaminants have been proven to cause cancer and other horrible illnesses, yet they are in our water supply! I was recently ridiculed by a family member for declining tap water at a restaurant, but clearly there is good reason. It is hard to think that in our "safe" country we have drinking water coming from the tap that is toxic and dangerous to our health. Most people probably never even think about it. Take a few minutes and check the database for your location. Then find the right filtration devices for your home.

I recommend you filter your water on the way into your house and before it gets to your cup or shower. Remember that chlorine will vaporize from your shower, your bath, your toilet and your washing machine and every other place you have a water tap, every time you use them! Asthma and allergies can worsen as can airway inflammation. These gases can build up in your home as well. EWG.org has a great guide to water filtration.

In addition to filtering your whole-house water and your drinking water, one fun thing to do is locate natural springs near your home and drink the water from them. The website www.findaspring.com is a nice way to locate natural springs near you. We have had several great family adventures finding natural springs and driving to them to get drinking water, and to enjoy their natural beauty. Teach your kids at an early age what clean and pure drinking water is, and how important it is to their health. [*]

---

[*] articles.mercola.com/sites/articles/archive/2017/08/08/toxins-found-in-public-tap-water.aspx

Endocrine disruptors in the bathroom

There are so many toxins in your bathroom!

Remember your skin will absorb everything you put on it, for better or for worse. Common chemicals like sodium lauryl sulfate, parabens, phthalates and triclosan, to name just a few, are very commonly added to personal care products such as body washes, regular shampoos, dry shampoos, lotions and body sprays. And those amazing and varied perfumed scents are laden with toxins. Even very expensive, and especially dermatologist-recommended products can be full of endocrine disruptors. Again, you may say, "These can't be toxic! They are dermatologist-recommended and so many people use them! Everyone uses scented products and regular soap and toothpaste! Why do they sell them if they aren't healthy?"

You have to be the one who is looking out for your health and for the health of your family. No government agency will ever take the place of individual consumer vigilance. Some simple things you can do in your bathroom and with your personal care products can potentially eliminate a continued toxic exposure. Use fabric shower curtains, not vinyl, which can gas off and be full of BPA. Stop using anti-bacterial soaps that contain triclosan, which is an endocrine disrupter. Basic soaps such as Dr. Bronner's or other castile-based soaps work just as well and do not hurt you in the process.

As much as you may love those fragranced soaps and lotions, those chemical fragrances are full of endocrine disruptors, as are your favorite perfumes! And think about where you spray these chemicals: right on your skin, even over your thyroid gland and other organs! Train your sense of smell (and you can!) to appreciate fragrances that are natural scents from fruits and flowers and herbs. I personally love lavender, and I make my own hand soap from unscented castile soap and lavender essential oils. I love making my own lotions and face creams as well, using only food grade products and essential oils for fragrance. You can find easy recipes on YouTube and Pinterest. They also make great gifts for family and friends.

Be aware that even though the label reads "natural" or "organic", the product may still contain phthalates or parabens. Also "perfume" or "fragrance" may be used to denote that the product has a specific scent, but if it is not marked as a natural fragrance or essential oil, they are more than likely endocrine disruptors.

Your cosmetics, including foundation, blusher, eye makeup and lipstick, often contain heavy metals and toxic chemicals. Recently, it was found that popular lipstick brands contain heavy metals such as lead.

EWG.org ranks many makeup companies, and you can see what chemicals are contained in your makeup or personal care item and the safety ranking listed for the individual product. This way you can test your favorite makeup brand and see what level of toxicity exists. You want the lowest number, like a number 1 or maybe 2, for your brand and product. The lower the number, the less toxicity. You may be very surprised and dismayed by how toxic common makeup and facial care brands are in the United States.

You will also be able to locate safe brands of makeup, lotions and facial care products at ewg.org. Several years ago, I was using a well-known, "natural" brand of facial care thinking I was doing a good job for myself. When someone told me about ewg.org, I entered in my facial wash and moisturizer, and the scoring came back as a 5 and 6. I was floored and did not want to believe it. As a result, I stopped using products that contained toxic substances and located a very safe, very nice, healthy alternative.

As a practitioner, I test patients' hormones on a regular basis. It is common that some hormone lab results come back showing extremely high levels of estrogen, testosterone or progesterone, for example. Many components are allowed into our personal care products and makeups that are not required to be listed on the ingredients list and are not regulated by the FDA at all. Often progesterone or other hormones, and even tissue from aborted fetuses, have been found in personal care products like "anti-aging" creams. Because of so much contamination in our personal care products especially of hormones that artificially skew results, one of my labs recently added a requirement that no lotions or makeups be used on the day of the sample collection. According to a piece on this topic at WebMD.com, "There is currently no limit on the amount of progesterone allowed in cosmetic products." * **

Be very cautious of buzz words like "anti-aging" or "youth". Sometimes after using these types of products and then being tested, levels of hormones show up in dangerously high amounts in the body. The hormone system is delicately balanced. To have extremely high amounts of any hormone in

---

* wb.md/2DAL3fP / bit.ly/2zMq6R3

** www.neocutis.com/corporate/ethical_commitment

the body increases the potential to imbalance the whole endocrine system. Using any type of hormone, including over-the-counter progesterone or DHEA for example, without the advice and help of a doctor or health professional can cause real damage to your body. It only takes a small amount of hormone to create very large changes. The last thing you want is to have dangerously high levels of harmful carcinogenic metabolites or estrogens coursing through your body. The symphony of your hormones will not be playing beautiful music if this is the case.

Too much of a good thing is not always good. There are rarely get-rich-quick schemes or lose-weight-quick schemes that don't take a toll somewhere on our bank accounts—or our bodies. A big problem we have in this country is the lack of transparency in labeling and the lack of oversight in what can be added to a personal care product, and what is required to be put on the label of that product. The side effects of these unknown ingredients can be very detrimental, and for most women, who are just trying to be beautiful or feel good, this knowledge can come as quite a shock.

I try to use the "less is more" motto when it comes to personal care products. I use very little makeup, and the products I use are ranked very low on EWG.org. I make use of essential oils and I do not use any perfumes at all. I use low-ranked shampoos, conditioners, deodorants, soap and hair color. No one is perfect, though, and we do not live in a perfect world. My changes took time to develop, and I still use some manufactured products that I know some women would never use, opting for even more natural substitutes.

You must decide for yourself how much you want to reduce in your life. Endocrine disruptors are everywhere. Can you find a healthier hair color that your colorist will use, or can you do it yourself with a healthier "at home" color?

Nail color is another source of endocrine disruptors that we need to be aware of. Do you get your nails done all the time or wait longer in between appointments? You could bring in your own nail color, minus the worst of the endocrine disruptors. Maybe you could only get your toes done in the summer when everyone sees them, or not at all.

I have friends who have opted to go completely gray rather than have any type of hair color. I have other friends who use hair color but try to minimize the toxins by finding ways to color roots more naturally in between colorings. I have used a more natural hair color at home myself for years now after I realized how toxic commercial hair colors are. Years ago, I used a commercial hair color that started a scalp dermatitis that spread to my face. After this experience, I realized my body could not tolerate commercial hair color.

Sunscreens are another place where we can take in endocrine disruptors into our body. Use organic and non-chemical sun screens as much as possible and use them as little as possible. Sunscreens are another product ranked on EWG.org so you can find a safe product there.

Reducing the levels of endocrine disruptors around the house, yard and garden

Take stock of your bathroom cleaners, floor cleaners, all-purpose cleaners and toilet bowl cleansers. I know I did not think of these things as toxic, but they are. These commercial cleaning products are full of poisons that are potent endocrine disruptors.

There are simple household cleaning products you can make with simple healthy ingredients such as vinegar, baking soda and lemons to clean your kitchen counters, windows and bathrooms, and stay safe yourself. There are also many products now being sold in stores that are safe and effective at cutting grease and sanitizing surfaces. You may be surprised at the power of vinegar to clean a dishwasher or baking soda to clean an oven. We have been so conditioned to using super toxic substances, where in many cases simplicity will do.

Other toxic substances that you may not be aware of are bug repellants, pesticides and herbicides. Pesticides and herbicides are xenoestrogens, which mimic the actions of estrogen in the body, wreaking all kinds of havoc. In the age of Zika and other bug-borne diseases, it is important to weigh risks and benefits. Again, EWG.org has abundant information on mosquito repellants and the safest ones for adults, children and pregnant women.

Endocrine disruptors in the yard

I am a gardener, and my specialty is organic vegetable gardening. I am the type of person who advocates for front yards and backyards as vegetable gardens, and side yards too, for that matter. I am a Cobb County Master Gardener and a member of Crossroads Community Garden. We garden organically, and though that is a challenge, to me it is the way things should be. I took an organic farming class a few years ago and I was privileged to learn from a female farmer who loves the earth and loves tending and cultivating the fruit of the ground, responsibly stewarding the earth in her possession. It was and is one of the best classes I have ever taken.

To be up early tending to the ground in the cool crisp winter, preparing the earth for planting, is one of life's pleasures for me. We planted potatoes in mounds, and constructed fencing and flapping fabric to keep the deer off our newly planted field. We planted vegetables in hoop houses for an early harvest and learned how to prepare seedlings for the spring planting. There were no bug sprays or harmful pesticides or Roundup sprayed on the plants. Cover crops like clover and alfalfa were planted in the fields to let the ground rest while other fields were prepared for planting.

There are very specific rules for organic farming, and the organic farmer must rotate crops from year to year so as not to use up the nutrients in the soils. Commercial farmers use up the nutrients in the soil by over-farming the ground year after year with the same crops, then replace the natural nutrients lost with chemical fertilizers. Soil is life, and the soils in our land are worn out and depleted just as we are. Farming and gardening organically is taking responsibility for our soils and our lands and our people. Spraying Roundup and other pesticides and herbicides has consequences.

We are killing off our honey bees and pollinators at an alarming rate, and insecticides have been determined to be the main cause of their demise. Insecticides, as the name indicates, kill insects, and when we kill insects, we often inadvertently kill pollinators. Pollinators are bees, bats, beetles and butterflies that carry pollen from plant to plant by collecting nectar. It is nature's way of reproducing, as pollen from the male part of the flower is moved to the female part, resulting in the production of fruits and seeds. Sometimes the wind moves pollen, but most often animals do that job very well.

Animals and insects in search of food move from plant to plant, feeding. Birds and butterflies move pollen on their bodies from one plant to another while they are feeding, while bees collect the pollen on purpose. When these animals collect pollen from a plant or flower sprayed or treated with insecticide, they die. When they die, the natural spread of pollen ceases and we are in big trouble.

Life without pollinators would be very bare indeed! There would be fewer berries and seeds and nuts, and fruits like blueberries and almonds would be gone. Vegetables like squash, as well as chocolates and coffee, would cease to exist. A world without chocolate and coffee? Over 75% of our flowering plants and crops are pollinated by these animals. Simply put, we cannot live without them!

The bottom line is if honey bees disappear we human beings will probably not go extinct, but our diets will be pretty boring. The California Almond Board says almonds "would not exist." Coffee bean flowers only open for pollination for three or four days. If there are no pollinators around during those days, there will be no coffee. Apples, onions, many types of berries and avocados rely on bees for pollination. If the population of honey bees and other pollinators decreases or disappears, our culinary delights will be severely limited. I do not want to think of life without these animals or life without these foods!

All our actions have consequences. Those massive amounts of pesticides and herbicides sprayed daily on our lawns and sidewalks in every subdivision across our country? We pay for that in honey bee and other pollinators' deaths and seepage of toxins into our ground water and into our water supplies. Why do we want signs in our yards warning pets and children to stay off the grass for fear of poisoning? If you have green grass, don't you want to walk and play on it safely?

It is a common occurrence to see the lawn trucks in my neighborhood with the pesticides being sprayed all over yards and sidewalks by men with backpacks of liquid death on their backs swinging their wands of liquid poison back and forth across the yards and green spaces. I fear for their health as well, walking around all day breathing in those fumes and spraying those toxins. But as usual it has been deemed "safe" and so we continue with our acres of grass blankets and industrial farms sown with the deaths of the very creatures that keep us all alive and give us variety in our diets and beauty in our world.[*] [**]

What can we do to save the pollinators? I have a few suggestions.

Buy organic seeds and plants, which are not treated with pesticides of any kind. Neonicotinoids are pesticides known to be deadly to bees. Make sure that any plant you buy from the big box stores or any nursery is not pre-treated with this insecticide. Stop using pesticides. The EPA lists 55 pesticides sold that contain neonicotinoid pesticides that are toxic to bees. These insecticides are not just harmful to bees; they are also harmful to humans.[***] [****]

My next suggestion is to plant an organic vegetable and pollinator garden. Use the space in your yard to grow lettuce and spinach and tomatoes and cucumbers—whatever your family enjoys eating. You can grow plants in pots or in raised beds or in the ground. It has been said that on just a quarter acre, enough food could be grown all year for a family of four.

Plant wild flowers in your yard. These will attract not only bees, but birds and other animals that further the pollination of plants. Pollinator plants attract butterflies of all kinds. My backyard is full of flowers for most of the growing season. I have butterflies and hummingbirds and all kinds of birds that nest and feed nearby.

Next, I suggest you make some native spaces in your landscaping. Most of us live under some type of covenant or Home Owner's Association. A few years ago, as I was living under such garden oppression, I grew a guerrilla vegetable garden in my front yard in direct violation of the "no visible garden or vegetable" rule because most people don't know a tomato from a weed. I grew a wild English type garden in the front yard in raised beds and pots and interspersed with the wild bushy flowers were rosemary and thyme and oregano and peppers and tomatoes and red okra.

I had purple trailing flowering vines growing up and over the tomato plants. The peppers just hid at the bottom, and everyone was so enamored of the beautiful blooms on that unusual plant (the red okra, which has

---

[*]   www.nrdc.org/onearth/would-world-without-bees-be-world-without-us

[**]   www.fws.gov/pollinators/

[***]   www.epa.gov/sites/production/files/2016-01/documents/infographic_jan._2016.pdf

[****]   www.epa.gov/pollinator-protection

unique flowers). I had summer onions growing with the petunias and I had the best time growing food in my front yard. Why this has become a sin punishable by fines dealt out by roving neighborhood spies who wander the neighborhoods staring into your private yards, I have no idea. We, however, sign the damnable neighborhood agreements, so I suppose we bear some responsibility for the aforementioned "no vegetable" decrees. I moved. Now I do not have the ubiquitous HOA in my neighborhood. I am much happier that way!

You can still make islands of pollinator plants and flowers in most front yards, even in restrictive covenant neighborhoods. You can grow herbs and other beautiful flowers that feed nature and give you beautiful visitors to view and visit with. Bees and other wildlife need places to nest and build homes. Having shrubby or weedy areas on your property can provide places of refuge and natural home sites for beneficial creatures.

Continuing the acres and acres of immaculate green pesticide carpets does not contribute much to the saving of the bees, or to the saving of mankind either for that matter, but to the contrary, are harming wildlife and human life. Just for the record, I am aware my lack of affinity for the manicured green space is not the most popular position. I would submit, however, that when you look at what is popular in many areas of life, it is often true that popularity does not coincide with conscience or even humanity.

Join the Million Pollinator Challenge, a campaign to register a million public and private gardens and landscapes to support pollinators.* Both of my gardens are registered. Go to pollinator.org and register your home or community garden if they are organic and refuges for pollinators.

If you do not have a garden, you can make one. Any garden store in your area would be happy to help you make a pollinator garden at your home or school or office.

Another great resource is The Master Gardener Program of which I am a proud member. This program, which consists of volunteers, is committed to educating the public about all aspects of gardening. Your county extension office will often have a Master Gardener available for free to answer questions about any and all kinds of gardening and farming.**

---

* millionpollinatorgardens.org

** *You can locate a Master Gardener at* articles.extension.org/mastergardener

Join a community garden. I first joined my community garden when I had too much shade to grow any vegetables in my back yard and the HOA didn't want me to use the front yard for a garden. It was at first a refuge and has grown to become a place of peace and joy for me where like-minded people join to grow vegetables to feed our families and the hungry in our community. My community garden donated hundreds of pounds of vegetables last year to Feed the Hungry. I can grow veggies wherever I want in my own yard now, but my community garden is a special place for me. You probably have one near you as well.

My opinion on pesticides and herbicides is that we should stop using them altogether. If you must have the perfect lawn, at least do some research and find non-toxic alternatives that will protect all of us from the voluntary spreading of endocrine disruptors in our midst. Your decisions on this could save humans and creatures alike. It starts with each of us making better decisions for ourselves and our children's future on this lovely planet.

Buying organic foods is the safest way to avoid pesticides and other endocrine disruptors in your vegetables and fruits. Organic meats and eggs are the only way to go to avoid antibiotics, drugs and other endocrine disruptors that are prevalent in the commercial meat industry.

Another common endocrine disrupter that no one really thinks about is grilled meat—that wonderful summer pastime that yields delicious and tender polycyclic aromatic hydrocarbons, or PAHs, which occur in charred meat. Many people genetically lack the ability to breakdown these endocrine disrupting toxins and open themselves up to these carcinogens building up in their bodies. Many of us should only consume one serving of smoked or grilled meat a week.

For more details on specific endocrine disruptors and insights into how to avoid them, visit www.globalhealingcenter.com/natural-health/hormonal-imbalance. Another site with a whole section on endocrine disruptors is EPA.gov.

The truth is that we live in a toxic world, and anything we can do to reduce the toxic load accumulating in our bodies will go a long way to protecting our delicate cell structures from endocrine disruptors. The key is to take one area of your life and improve it a little. Then take the next area. Try not to get overwhelmed with how much is wrong, but rather look at one area you can improve, then move to the next. Over the years, I have developed strategies for dealing with many different aspects of toxicities, but it did not happen overnight.

The book *Living Healthy in a Toxic World*, written by David Steinman and R. Michael Wisner, is a wonderful resource, and gives you simple ways to protect yourself and your family from toxins and poisons in our world today.

We can make a difference. It seems impossible, but it's not. And the difference, as it is with so many things, is education. Start by educating yourself. Then teach your family and your friends and so on. When we all see and understand what is going on in our world we can demand, and then create, a cleaner, saner world.

For more information, visit the following links:

www.rmichaelwisner.com/human-detoxification/the-solution/

www.globalhealingcenter.com/natural-health/hormonal-imbalance/

clearbodyclearmind.com

CHAPTER 12
The Body Electric

"MAGIC'S JUST SCIENCE THAT WE DON'T UNDERSTAND YET."

– ARTHUR C. CLARKE

Your body has an energy field; this is a fact, borne out by recent studies. As technology advances we will see more and more that the things that cannot be seen are there working for us whether we believe it or not. Many people are not aware of this research and believe there is no such thing as an energy field around the body, and science, not having objective ways to measure it, has often denied its presence.*

Many medical doctors and even some alternative practitioners poo-poo the idea that the body has energy that runs through and around it, and that healing and information can be obtained from this area of the body. Chinese medicine has relied for over 5000 years on the Chi, or the energy of the body. Acupuncture has brought relief and healing to millions of people, and this practice is based on the excess or deficiency of this energy called Chi.

In all forms of healing there are names for energy: Prana and Ki are just two others. The practitioners of martial arts and other healing methods are very familiar with this energy. The energy that is emitted from the hands of these practitioners can be measured, and focusing it into the hands or other body parts can play a very significant role—both in healing and the martial arts.

Medicine and science have long been skeptical of anything not easily seen or measured. When I first saw this method of testing using the body's energy field, I too was skeptical. It did not seem real. How could someone tell what was going on with a body by testing the energy field? But on the other hand, if just a small percentage of what I was seeing was real, we were really onto something.

---

* www.reiki.org/reikinews/sciencemeasures.htm

It was only when I became ill that I had the experience that would ultimately change the course of my career. Energy is a fleeting thing. It changes and flows. It has a message for us if only we know how to ask and how to listen. I have become very adept at both asking and listening.

Your body has a story to tell. The body is alive. It is not a stone or a piece of brick. It has life, and because of this it has an intelligence. That intelligence runs our body and tells it what to do every day without our input or interference. This is the intelligence that created our bodies while we grew inside our mothers.

We did not have to stop daily and tell the body what to do, what organ to grow next, what bone needed to be built. Nine months later, a new life came into the world without anyone consciously doing any of the construction. So, I need to ask you the question: if the body can do this, why do we have such a tough time understanding that it can heal itself?

Why do we struggle on and on with illness, taking pill after pill, enduring surgery after surgery? Why don't we use the information and the intelligence of the body to access data that can help us heal? I have seen day after day, in patient after patient, the beauty of the body. I work with the energy field, with the basic nutritional needs of the body and with functional and conventional labs to give me hard and important data about the internal physiological processes and specific hormone outputs of the body.

What I tell my patients, and what I will tell you, is that this is not a "belief system". Whether you "believe" or "don't believe", the body will still march on. Your energy field still exists. If you want to be well, if you eat well and do the things necessary to heal, you will heal. Your heart will beat, your liver will filter toxins, your colon will move waste through your body, your nervous system continues to control your body, belief or not.

Muscle reflex testing is using the body's own energetic mechanisms to access information regarding the body systems of an individual for use in developing a natural health program for that person. The use of a testing muscle can enable the practitioner to communicate with the intelligence of the body to locate stresses, and possible underlying causes, that can then be backed up with lab testing. This allows us multiple windows into the healing possibilities that exist in the body. With these vital pieces of information, a detailed and individualized health program can be created, enabling the patient to move from sickness and ill health to wellness.

The fact that one can test the body through the energy field is demonstrated to me daily at my clinic. I test the body energetically and often find stresses in the body systems. These may include areas of pain or malfunction, areas of deficiencies or organ stress. As I said before, though, energy can be fickle. I have learned to work with this and to make my testing as accurate as possible, taking into consideration the fluctuations and changes of the energy field around the body. I have developed systems to check myself and those I am testing as well, so I can move accurately through the ebb and flow of the energy that can and does tell us so much.

Our energetic reflex testing is designed to give clues about possible stresses and to ask the body's opinion, if you will, about what is going on. A skilled muscle tester can often tell you more about what is happening in your body than you could ever imagine. Back in the early 90s, a friend of mine sent me a VHS video of muscle testing. I watched it and was fascinated. I was also very "science based" and "evidence based", and I was very skeptical. I do remember thinking, though, that if what this teacher was saying was even remotely true this could help a lot of people.

In the end, my skepticism won out and I thought the video was a joke and that I would be laughed out of town if I took this seriously. I threw the tape into a drawer.

Fast forward to my own serious health condition a few years later. My medical providers told me I had to have surgery, and when I dared question them on alternatives and asked to pursue another opinion, I was fired as a patient!

This left me scared, with a serious health problem and no doctor. When I sought alternative options, I learned from an amazing doctor in upstate Minnesota that there were ways to access the energy field of the body to get information. He used acupuncture points and a computer that read many different areas of stress. This was my first experience with an alternative healing practice other than chiropractic, and I was surprised and very humbled to realize how much I did not know. This wonderful healer helped me understand that what I ate and the elevated toxin levels in my body were very much to blame for what was happening to me medically.

He could access information about what was going on in my body that none of my medical doctors back home were able to do. They did not know how to access this information. But this doctor was in Minnesota, so I had to find someone closer to home to help me. On my return, I found a doctor in North Georgia and made an appointment.

Now here, my friends and possible skeptics, is where I found that I had a guiding hand on my path. As I walked into this doctor's office, lo and behold—what should be playing on the television but the same video I had received from my friend a couple of years earlier! The same one I had watched in fascination and then in skepticism. The same one that was still in that bottom drawer of my desk at work. You know that moment when you realize that someone's been trying to tell you something and if you'd listened—well you get the picture. I had to get sick to become humble enough to hear what was being said.

I was tested using this muscle reflex testing technique and was told exactly what my doctor had told me in Minnesota, and even more information that was extremely accurate to my current health condition. I was astonished! I was given a liver detox, a very specific treatment plan and some strict diet instructions, and the path to my own healing and my practice transformation began.

Shortly after, I began taking continuing education classes to learn these advanced alternative healing techniques myself, for use in my own practice, and to become an expert in the body's energy field. I too wanted to communicate with the body itself to derive information and data to help people get well from all kinds of illnesses. I had so many patients I needed to help. At this point in my career I started on the road to becoming a healer—or in my mind a "real doctor".

For the first time, I could tell a patient I could help them with menstrual cramps, with feelings of exhaustion and with digestive distress. I am a doctor who seeks the real reasons behind an illness; who looks for underlying causes, not quick fixes. I am a doctor who takes time to listen and who sincerely cares about her patients. A doctor who will never give up and always, always holds hope and space for healing for her patients. I am a doctor who asks questions about diet and lifestyle and is willing to give the correct information and advice whether it is easy to deliver or not.

A doctor who knows healing is not in my hands but in the hands of the person sitting in front of me.

This has been my chosen path now for well over twenty years. Using my muscle response testing to give me the body's take on the situation, my heart rate variability testing to give me a check and balance on the nervous system, and my functional and conventional lab testing to find the true causes behind health issues, I have been solving puzzles and putting the pieces of my patients' health right again for thousands of patients. I am grateful to be the coach, to be the person my patients have chosen to help them become well, sometimes for the first time in their lives. It is an honor for me to be an instrument of healing for others.

I love to solve problems of the body. I love the endocrine system and the beautiful way that all the systems of the body work together to achieve balance. I love the order of the hormones and the function of the organs themselves and the fact that the body works with us to be well, not against us. I love how the digestive system can be made right again, even after tremendous stress and damage, if the right steps are taken to heal it. Putting order back into the chaos that can be created in the body is what I do best. For me, talking to a body is like shaking hands with an old friend.

The body will divulge its secrets, which are not actually secrets, as they live right there on the surface for anyone to find if only they ask the right questions. With reflex testing, I can tell you how you probably feel at certain times of the day and what symptoms might be bothering you. I can scan for potential stresses, sensitivities or possible toxicities in the body. I can begin to look for the causes behind your health concerns. I can start the conversation towards wellness with your body.

The things we cannot see are sometimes the things that matter most to us. You cannot see love, but you can feel it. You cannot see hate, but you know it's there. You cannot see God, but for many he is present. As Arthur C. Clarke said, "Magic's just science that we don't understand yet."

There is much that we humans do not understand fully. I have learned this through my own illness and healing, through the fire of my oldest son's illness and subsequent healing, through alternative and energy medicine, through the thousands of patients I have been privileged to work with over the years. I do know, though, that my gift is in knowing what is true and what will be helpful for the body on its path back to wellness. Knowing this, I can give the body a blueprint for what it needs to get back to health, back to better balance.

Can you guess at this point the energy technique that identified a formula for my infant son when he was so sick and unable to hold anything down? That enabled us to find foods he could tolerate that let him grow again? That enabled me to help his poor sick little body get well and grow into the fine man he is today? Yes, the technique that gave us the initial clue to the underlying causes of his health issues and a path to its eventual solution was muscle reflex testing.

My hope for all of us, especially in this country, is that we do not allow our hubris to keep us from seeking and finding the solutions that could help us if only we could suspend our disbelief for a moment, and simply do the things that work—even if they defy conventional thought. It matters what we eat, what we think and who we are connected to in our personal and business lives. It matters what toxins are in our food and our water. Fixing these things can really make a huge difference—sometimes the difference between life and death. Often, the simple things are the best things— listening, caring, doing what makes sense for the patient, not the insurance carrier or the drug companies or the special interests.

There is joy and magic in the human body if only we allow it to be well.

Following is a link to a widely known and patented muscle-testing technique by Yoshiaki Omaura, MD, ScD, FACA, FICAI, DAAPM, FAAIM, FRSM:

www.bdort.org

CHAPTER 13
Evectics^{SM}: An Entirely New Approach to Health Care

"IF YOU ONLY HAVE A HAMMER,
YOU TEND TO SEE EVERY PROBLEM AS A NAIL."

– ABRAHAM MASLOW

With every case, I am targeting causal agents and formulating a program that leads to better health and overall positive outcomes for the patient. I create a very specific individualized program that enables someone to move from sick and tired to healthy and well, full of energy, vitality and focus!

I have developed a technique that enables me to do this. It is called **Evectics^{SM}**.

This health improvement technique, which I developed, adapts to every aspect of the individual case. This completely customized approach is a radical departure from traditional and alternative medicine techniques.

In the 1800s, the word "evectics" (*e-VEK-tics*) meant "The branch of medical science which teaches the method of acquiring a good habit of body." In other words, evectics meant "the method of obtaining health." The word went out of use in the early 1900s, as medicine became more about relief of symptoms and less about health. I have resurrected it as a name for my system of individualized health improvement therapy.

How Evectics differs from traditional medicine

To help you understand this new technology, I will give you a comparison between Evectics and traditional medicine's handling of chronic health problems.

Evectics: testing, understanding, and *then* therapy

When we first start with you as a patient we test you. Decades of experience with difficult cases has taught me that anything can happen in a case, and that I must test thoroughly before any therapy is even planned.

Rather than test just the areas associated with your complaint, I test to determine why your body cannot heal. This is fundamentally different from the medical approach, which is based on symptoms (including symptoms that show up on labs: your blood test values are symptoms, they are not causing the health problems that created them).

Once I know which areas of your body are stressed and the cause of that stress, your entire case history, current and past symptoms and other factors that can affect healing, I'm ready to choose the specific tools required in your case and create a customized program.

This is a dramatic departure from other medical and alternative approaches to diagnosis and treatment.

Evectics uses individualized therapy

Your body needs the treatment it needs, even if your doctor only knows how to do something else.

It is completely amazing to me that this isn't obvious to everyone else.

If you go to:

- A **medical doctor**, you will in all likelihood leave with a prescription for a drug.

- A **chiropractor**, you will almost certainly receive a chiropractic adjustment.

- A **nutritionist**, you will probably get a recommendation for supplements and vitamins.

- An **acupuncturist**, you'll get an acupuncture treatment.

- A **naturopath**, you will often get lab and supplement recommendations.

You will receive a treatment based on what the doctor you happen to go to knows how to do, not based on what your body may need to heal.

In many cases, patients are "going to a plumber for an electrical problem" but don't realize this, because the plumber tells them he can fix their wiring.

Bodies with complex problems often need many different types of treatment.

This is one reason your chronic problem may change somewhat under conventional or alternative treatment, but never resolve. Your treatment with a doctor may not be incorrect, but if you are under only one type of treatment when your body needs several, you will get incomplete results at best.

The Evectics toolkit

Following is a list of some of the Evectics tools. While not a complete list, it will give you an idea of some of the main tools I use:

- **CLINICAL NUTRITION** Exact dietary supplements based on ongoing testing. There are four major divisions of this technique: whole food and therapeutic supplementation, drainage remedies, homeopathy and herbology.

- **SDT—SYSTEMS DESENSITIZATION TECHNIQUE** An acupressure technique (no needles, we use cold laser to stimulate the acupuncture points) to help the body recover from allergies, sensitivities, immune and inflammation issues and gut and digestive stress.

- **SBT— SYSTEMS BALANCING TECHNIQUE** An acupressure technique (nine specific protocols) to help the body recover from hormone imbalances caused by toxins in the food and environment.

- **DIET/LIFESTYLE** My program is focused on improving immune response, not just "eating healthy." This approach can result in rapid improvement of a patient's problems as well as long-term health benefits.

- **CRAVINGS SOLUTIONS** Acupressure therapies to put you back in control of what you eat.

- **HEART RATE VARIABILITY (HRV)** Computerized testing of the autonomic nervous system (the private network that the body uses to run itself—digesting food, growing hair, healing, etc.) to identify and resolve nervous system problems that can prevent or slow the healing process.

- **FUNCTIONAL LAB TESTING** Most people are very familiar with diagnostic testing, which is often blood labs they get from their doctor. These labs show symptoms (high cholesterol, for example) that can be suppressed with a drug or other values high or low that indicate a possible problem. A different approach to lab testing is functional labs, tests of blood, saliva, hair, urine and stool that are designed to give the doctor information related to how the body is functioning. This information, when used with other forms of testing and observing how the body responds to various therapies, can provide objective information on what tools the doctor should use and what approach the body will respond to and work with.

An Evectics practitioner has a full set of tools, not just one treatment method, and can use accurate testing and case programming to know exactly which tools to use, in what combination and in what order. This is a very important key to resolving chronic health problems.

The medical opinion

"One accurate measurement is worth a thousand expert opinions."

– Adm. Grace Hopper

Evectics uses testing, not opinion.

When medical doctors are treating chronic health conditions, they often rely largely on their opinion of what is wrong and what treatment is needed. This is so true that it's normal to seek a "second opinion" to see if you can get more than one doctor to agree on your treatment.

My view is that measurement and testing should replace opinion. An opinion is really a guess.

Using accurate testing to determine what therapies the body needs and in what order they are required is called "case programming".

Correct, effective case programming based on accurate testing is crucial.

A well-done case program correctly interprets the testing and labs and does not rely on the doctor's experience or opinion. The case program is a step-by-step written guide to resolving the patient's case.

Evectics practitioners are specifically trained in case programming and use exact testing instead of guesswork.

Practitioners operate with the help of a highly-trained case director who checks programs, patient progress (quality control) and consults with practitioners.

Patient progress is surveyed and measured at every visit, analyzed and graphed to find any slowdowns or inefficiencies and if they are found, a plan is made to resolve them.

Finish your Evectics program with good, stable health and live a wellness lifestyle!

When are you done with a treatment program?

A question I often ask of doctors (both medical and alternative) is, "When do you know that your patient is done with their treatment program?" Here are a few answers I hear regularly:

- When they feel better and don't want to come in anymore.

- When I have completed the standard treatment protocol (often regardless of outcome).

- When their insurance runs out.

- If they don't respond well to my treatment, I refer them to a specialist.

None of these answers have much to do with regaining a stable state of health.

Three goals of an Evectics treatment program

Here are three goals for a sensible treatment program that has as its aim the restoration of health rather than control of symptoms:

- The patient's body is no longer a problem in his or her life.

- The patient is not worried or anxious over what could happen to his or her health in the future.

- The patient feels confident in his own knowledge and ability to maintain good health through a lifestyle from now on.

With these goals achieved to the satisfaction of the patient, the patient can be successfully graduated from a treatment program and monitored occasionally a few times a year on a wellness program to catch and head off any developing health issues.

An Evectics program is complete when the patient is satisfied with the results and tests show the improvements are stable.

And it works!

During two decades of research and testing, I have helped patients' bodies to heal almost every type of health problem.[*]

Clinical nutrition and muscle reflex testing

Muscle reflex testing is a technique using muscle biofeedback originally developed by Dr. George Goodheart in the 1950s. His work led to the development of Applied Kinesiology, which is taught in schools and used by doctors across the world. Using this technique, the practitioner tests the strength of an "indicator muscle" such as the deltoid.

To use the deltoid as an indicator muscle, the patient extends an arm at a right angle to the body. The practitioner tests the strength of the muscle by pushing down on the arm from the patient's wrist. Then the practitioner can do any number of actions designed to test whether a substance or area of the body causes stress to the nervous system. If the action causes stress, the arm weakens. No stress, the arm stays strong.

Implicit in all my techniques is the concept of helping the body regain its ability to heal. If a patient has a problem that would be successfully resolved with traditional medicine, the answer to the question *What is the cause of this problem?* would lead to a medical diagnosis and medical treatment.

If the problem is chronic and the cause is a deterioration of the body's ability to heal, then often no medical treatment would resolve the problem other than to relieve symptoms, if it did that. In this case, the correct question to ask would be *What obstacle is there to healing?* The answer to this question opens the door to possible ways to assist the body back to a state of healing and health.

Assisting the body to regain its health relies on accurate and current information on what the body needs now. Functional lab testing can provide background information and key facts and clues to help see directly into the body's biological functions. Even more effective are techniques that

---

[*] *You can find hundreds of testimonials from patients at* alternativehealthatlanta.com/ testimonials/.

help the body heal utilizing current, real-time information directly from its own intelligence.

This information is uniquely available in the autonomic nervous system ("ANS"), which is the private network the body uses to control itself. The information available is, however, quite basic. I can't ask *What should I do?* and get a detailed answer. The ANS report is limited to varying degrees of stress, the location and cause of the stress. It can also differentiate among many sources of stress to report which has the priority, which would be the stress the body is currently stuck on, the stress that must be reduced for the body to continue to make progress toward healing.

All this information is available in the ANS; what's needed is a way to access it by testing.

Autonomic Response Evaluation ("ARE")

In the past twenty years of clinical experience and research, I have further refined the application of these basic scientific principles, and I call my technique Autonomic Response Evaluation, or ARE. Familiarity with this type of testing is not common, and the patients I've talked to who had heard about it still had no real understanding of how it works. What follows is a basic explanation.

1. The patient extends an arm, and the practitioner tests that the deltoid muscle is strong by pushing down on it.

2. The practitioner takes an action designed to test a specific area or item as a stress to the body. For example, the practitioner could apply pressure to an acupuncture point associated with a specific organ, such as the heart.

3. With the body's attention focused on the heart by way of pressure on the heart point, the practitioner applies force to the arm.

4. If the heart reflex is stressing the body, this stress will cause a stimulation to the Golgi tendon organ reflex in the deltoid muscle as it is being stressed by the practitioner's push, and the muscle will weaken, causing the arm to drop.

5. The Golgi tendon organ reflex is a protective reflex designed to prevent muscles from tearing tendons by making the muscle weak.

6. If the heart reflex isn't stressed, no stimulation to the Golgi tendon organ reflex will occur, and the arm will stay strong.

7. Other stresses put inside the body's energy field can be tested in a similar way. For example, a food can be placed on the body to determine with testing if that food might be stressful to the body.

Acupressure therapies

We use two proprietary acupressure therapies in my office. The Systems Desensitization Technique is used to help the body to be more tolerant of nutrients and utilize them better. It also can make the body less reactive to items like foods and environmental allergens when exposed to them in everyday life. We have seen this technique enable hundreds of people to add more foods back into their diet where once they could not eat them, and many can now face the allergy seasons without extreme discomfort and distress.

This technique has been life changing for many. Imagine being able to eat and enjoy foods you never thought you would be able to consume, and enjoying the outdoors when previously you could not even venture out during pollen season. If you suffer from allergies or sensitivities of any kind, this technique may be the answer you have been looking for.

In fact, the technique saved my son's life. In the deepest days of his sickness, this technology allowed us to find food which he was able to eat safely and grow.

This is a very simple and painless therapy, but very powerful. I use specific acupressure points, often enabling the body to better tolerate the allergen or sensitivity it is dealing with.

I need to add here that not everyone can benefit in this way. There are many factors that need to be taken into consideration, in every case, for someone to do this safely. Especially if one has an anaphylactic reaction to foods, extreme caution must be used by practitioners to ensure the patient's safety.

In the second type of therapy, Systems Balancing Technique, we use acupressure points to direct the body to normalize or balance certain organs that are directly responsible for hormone activity. You want to have balanced hormone activity and organs that work properly. As discussed in

Chapter 4, endocrine disruptors contribute to extreme hormone imbalance in today's world.

Using this technique enables me to open the body's drainage organs, and as a result increase its ability to clear out toxins and to balance the endocrine organs responsible for healthy hormone activity. As in all areas of the body, when we remove obstacles and areas of stress the body can heal and operate at a higher level of health.

These two techniques enable the body to operate at a higher functional level. In doing so, they open the door to healing.

Lab testing

There are many ways to test the body. I use what are termed functional labs in addition to the labs that you may be familiar with through your medical physical examinations. These functional labs test body function, not just values. For example, knowing what a hormone level is at one time is often important, but seeing how that hormone changes over the course of the day can be even more valuable.

In my clinic, we look at blood labs, stool labs, urine labs and saliva labs, to name a few. These labs are determined based on history and presenting health goals. With the information that muscle testing gives us, added to the patient history and lab results, we have a very nice picture from several angles, of what is going on in the body.

Working with energy is beautiful and challenging, as the body is always changing. I run both conventional and functional labs to pinpoint specific stresses the body may be experiencing, so I can enhance the body's own healing capabilities. I run labs specifically designed so that something can be done about the findings. I do not test just to generate pages and pages of information that may not be useful at all.

My goal is to enable the body to become the best that it can be. I do not treat or diagnose anything. I know the important things that a body needs to be well, and I work to give these things to the body in front of me. Health and wellness have many prerequisites. A happy, positive attitude and disposition is very important. We have discussed clean eating and good sleep. There are specific nutrients and hormone levels that make a body function better.

Some people's bodies are too far gone, and some do not possess the right attitude for healing. But if you want to be well, if you are willing to eat, sleep and move in a healthy manner and learn to understand how your body functions, and you want a plan to get there, I can help you. I have seen with thousands of patients that if you do everything in your power to be well, with the right tools and guidance the body's healing potential is amazing.

Some of the necessary labs I run at my office show specific functional stresses on different organs. Adrenal stress can cause adrenal fatigue, and action on this is a top priority. When the adrenals function at optimum, your body will function that much better. These types of functional labs enable me to see the functioning of an organ, not just a level that is either in or out of the normal range.

Knowing for sure if you are allergic to a food or other substance is invaluable. There are many allergies or sensitivities that are delayed, and one cannot pinpoint exactly where the reaction may have begun. Deficiencies in vitamins and minerals are very common in our world today. Knowing exactly what these are can enable us to put you on the correct supplementation program designed specifically for you.

As every body is different, yours needs what you need. Time and time again I have seen proof that an individualized health program designed just for you will give you the best results in the long term. Specific lab testing plays a key role in not only locating the problem but in tracking progress and results.

Some of the most important labs I look at are hormone labs. The functional adrenal labs and the female hormone labs contain vital information that help us understand the stress the body has been under and the damage that has been caused as a result. In reading basic blood chemistry, stool or urine labs, hormone labs and tests that show nutrient deficiency, I can piece together essential information on each case and see causative elements and functional deficiencies that can lead to specific and individualized programs and an overall resolution of a case, resulting in increased health.

Over the last several years, genetic testing and new technology have enabled me to be even more specific in my patients' care. We all know we are different from one another, but what does that mean and how do these differences affect us? What do those differences look like in our bodies?

Are you an extremely sensitive person who struggles all the time with your health, watching everything you eat, while your friends seem to be able to eat anything and never get sick? There are reasons for that, and often we can see them in your genetics.

I use an amazing genetic test in my practice that lets me see on a genetic level, often like a crystal ball, what your future health has in store for you. This test can give you that "edge" you may have been looking for.

Would you like to know if you are really "salt sensitive", information that is very valuable if you have blood pressure issues? Contrary to common belief, not everyone is sensitive to salt. Would you like to know the "best" exercise for your body, be it aerobics or biking or weight training, or the best combination? Would you like to know exactly how much calcium or B vitamins or vitamin D you need for your best health? Would you like to know if you have highly functioning detox capabilities to rid the body of toxins and poisons, or if your systems are deficient in this area? How about knowing if you can absorb calcium and vitamin D in optimum quantities to prevent osteoporosis? Or do you have a propensity for developing diabetes or high cholesterol?

All of these and more can be determined by your very own genetic test. The test I use examines at least 45 genetic markers that give us a picture of your current lifestyle your existing genetics and where the weaknesses are in your nutritional needs. This can help you plan for the rest of your life! We can begin now to protect your cardiovascular system, increase your chances of avoiding diabetes and other "inherited" conditions, because with knowledge comes power and with this power you can make yourself well.

That is why I love to do these tests. Of course, we all have the genetics we received from our parents, but do we have to express all the genes we were born with? Do we have to have all the things our parents had health wise? Are we just helpless and waiting for the inevitable to come? My answer is a resounding "NO!" The relatively new study of Epigenetics speaks about the reality that we have much more of a say about our genetic future than perhaps we have been led to believe.

Epigenetics is founded on the principle that environment and lifestyle choices and behaviors, and even stress and emotional reactions, can change the genetic outcomes of our current lives and even those of our offspring. Geneticists have observed that these factors can "flip an on-and-off switch" for genes that can determine a multitude of illnesses and even cancers.

For instance, the people we choose to be around, the joy we find in our lives, the love we create, the choices we make in choosing optimism or pessimism all play a role in our genetic expression. This fascinating fact suggests that if we can create these things for ourselves, we may have more control than we thought over what our genetics can and do express. It is a liberating thought! We are more in control of our bodies and their future health outcomes when we create healthy physical and mental habits.

Bioidentical hormones

Perimenopause and menopause are special times in a woman's life. It is sometimes hard for us to realize that our bodies are not still twenty-two! I know I do not feel my age. The truth is, though, that our bodies are not the same after forty as they were when we were twenty, nor should they be, they have been and will continue to change throughout our lives.

As my goal is to look at the function of the body's systems, my programs are directed towards healing and increasing the function of organ systems and the body as a whole. When hormones are replaced in the body, naturally or not, the body picks up on the levels, measuring them and notifying other body parts to release more or less hormones, depending on the amounts present in the tissues. It stands to reason, in my way of looking at it, that we need to fix the function of organs as much as possible so that the body can handle its own hormone output.

I have found that many women, for example, are suffering with adrenal fatigue that is making all their symptoms much worse. Addressing this and assisting the adrenal glands to heal and regain function can in many cases allow a woman's body to create the correct amount of female hormones that she needs to be healthy without adding more—even bioidentical ones—to her body systems.

A great deal has been written about bioidentical hormones, so let's take a closer look at them.

By *bioidentical*, I mean hormones that are chemically structured like the naturally occurring hormones found in the body. Drug companies chemically alter the hormones in conventional hormone replacement therapies, so they can patent them and sell them. These alterations are often responsible for harmful side effects, and as a result, they are endocrine disruptors.

The hormone system of our bodies is so delicately balanced that it does not take much to imbalance it. For this reason, I do not give a woman even a bioidentical hormone supplement without testing her body beforehand to determine her current levels of hormones. The testing of female hormones is still a developing technology, and not every practitioner is skilled and competent at this. It is wise to find a provider who tests the body first and does frequent follow-up testing after the initial recommendation of bioidentical hormones to make sure the body is responding well to the therapy.

I cannot tell you the number of women I have seen who have been put on conventional hormone treatment and bioidentical hormone treatment and have never been tested afterwards—even once—to see if the levels are too high or too low! This is dangerous, and in my opinion negligent care. If you choose to use bioidentical hormones, I urge you to find someone to work with who will test your adrenal status as well as other blood levels such as blood sugar, cholesterol, vitamin D and other important lab values that are vital to your health.

In addition, work with someone who understands that the function of organs and healing of the body as a whole is more important than just replacing hormones that seem to be deficient. A healthy and normally functioning body will handle many of its own problems!

During this time in your life, your female hormones and your body are changing in ways that can sneak up on you if you are not careful. As hormone levels decrease, bone density can decrease, cholesterol can increase, and fat percentages can rise. As a result, blood pressure and sugar levels can go up, and these changes now make us as prone to heart disease as our male counterparts.

Before menopause we are protected by our hormone levels, and these magical hormones make us much less likely to have heart problems at a young age. Now that we are in menopause and even perimenopause, however, we need to be aware that as these hormone levels drop we must take very specific precautions for our current and future health. I don't mean to scare you, but I do want you to be concerned. Osteoporosis, late stage diabetes, strokes, heart disease and a poor quality of life are not ideal outcomes to a life well lived! We have the tools now to prevent these chronic conditions and starting now is the key to a better future and high quality of life as you age.

I use several different labs to test hormone levels for the adrenals and female hormones.

- I use blood labs to make sure blood chemistry, cholesterol levels, inflammation levels and triglycerides are normal.
- I track blood sugar and blood pressure.
- I test for metabolites that show if bone tissue is breaking down faster than it is building up.
- I test for vitamin D, vitamin B and iodine levels.
- I use thermography testing for breast health.
- I test genetics for basic strengths and weaknesses.
- I test for basic mineral needs and imbalances
- I test for hormonal imbalance

Based on the results of these tests and other findings, I put together a program specifically and individually for each woman, so she knows all these issues are being addressed appropriately.

If you are a woman in the perimenopause or menopause stage of life, you might do your own personal health assessment and see if you are in need of some additional self-care. If so, take care of yourself now and find a professional to help you.

You can find hundreds of testimonials from patients at:

alternativehealthatlanta.com/testimonials/

CHAPTER 14
Now It's Up to You: Take Charge and Take Action!

Your life and health are in your hands. I hope that you can see that there is hope and that something can be done about many of your health problems. I hope that as you read this book you received some encouragement and some ideas to make your life and your health a bit better, or even a lot better. I am often asked by women, "What can be done for me?" or "Can you help me?" These are questions that can only be answered by gathering more information and understanding your specific health needs. There are a couple of ways I can help.

If you have a health problem, I would love to hear from you to see if I could assist you in some way. If you would like to travel to my office, as many people do, we can help you arrange logistics for your stay in our area and your appointments here at our office so you can get the most out of your visit. Ideally, you should arrange to be at our office for at least four or five days for your first visit. So much can be accomplished in a short time to get you more stable, and we usually see patients back at my office on subsequent visits based on their own personal circumstances.

It can be hard for someone from a conventional medical background to appreciate that there are effective methods of handling the body apart from drugs and surgery. If you think about it, unless the surgery is for a life-threatening illness or injury, it is often performed because of the failure of the doctor or provider to resolve the problem at hand. Please remember that the only thing that is responsible for healing is the body's own resilience. What I do at my office is to increase the body's own healing potential, allowing it to get back into the driver's seat and heal itself.

When you come to my office for the first time, we can quickly assess what obstacles your body is facing in healing, and we make a start at removing these and educating you as well, so that you can care for your body better! I have had patients come to my practice from out of town and rent a condo for several months at a time to receive care that will make their bodies stable. I have also had people come for a few days or a week and make subsequent visits, while we maintained progress using Skype and phone consults on a regular basis.

I have worked with patients outside the country by Skype and phone. If you would like to have a consultation with me by phone to see if I can help you, please call Alternative Health Atlanta at 770-937-9200. We will take your information and schedule a phone consultation. There are some who cannot travel to me and whom I may not be able to help long distance, because of the complexity of the case or any number of reasons. For these precious ladies I have written the following so that you can find an alternative practitioner in your area and get help. It is most important to me that you find help somewhere with someone that can guide you to making the best healthcare decisions.

How to find a practitioner in your area

My office, Alternative Health Atlanta, is in the city of Marietta, a few miles north of Atlanta, Georgia. We are happy to help you by phone or Skype if travel here is not an option for any reason. In my experience, however, there are some health problems that need a one-on-one relationship in a local setting with a qualified health specialist or practitioner. I am often asked how to find a good, qualified alternative health practitioner in a particular area. Here are some things I look for when trying to locate a health provider for myself or someone else.

First and foremost, the provider must have the philosophy that the body can heal itself and they must be specifically looking for the underlying root cause of a health problem. You can see this information on a website or by calling the front desk and asking the receptionist about the doctor or practitioner's practice. You can often have a consultation with the practitioner by phone or in person before you start a program. I think this is a good way to assess your compatibility with the person you will be working with.

All practices and doctors are different. There are many paths of training and clinical experiences and just searching key words like "alternative" or "functional" or "holistic" does not ensure you will find a doctor who has the training and experience needed in your case.

Many types of professionals can be alternative practitioners. These include, DCs (chiropractors) DOs (osteopaths) MDs (medical doctors) NPs (nurse practitioners) LAcs (acupuncturists), NDs (naturopaths), and other types of holistic practitioners.

You can search for alternative treatment, clinical nutrition, holistic therapy, functional medicine and many others. Twenty-five years ago, alternative healthcare was new and not really known. I could count on the fingers of one hand the number of alternative doctors in our area at that time. Now, many practices of all professions want to be "alternative", so you must know what you are looking for in a doctor or professional. Just treating someone with some "remedies" or giving a couple of supplements for "wellbeing" may be helpful, but these are not in-depth or experienced alternative or functional practitioners.

When you Google a practitioner, use the key word you are searching for and your area. It is important to read what is available online about the practice and the doctor, how they operate and what type of work they do specifically. Even better, get a referral from a friend or someone you trust. It is always better to go to a practitioner for whom you have received a positive referral. If there is a website, read it and look at training and experience. If the person has written a book, read it. Facebook, Twitter, YouTube and blogs are all places to gather information about a doctor or an office.

Specifically, you are looking for someone who understands the human body and how to utilize diet, functional labs, specific supplementation such as whole food supplements, herbal supplements, homeopathic remedies and possibly some type of energy therapy for healing and rebuilding purposes. Most offices will specialize in a specific type of health issue like hormone issues, musculoskeletal problems, blood sugar issues etc.

A website is often a great place to determine if the doctor seems knowledgeable and has experience with alternative health solutions for the issues you may be experiencing. Do you like the doctor's philosophy? Do you feel you could follow the program they have at the office you are looking at? For example, some programs stress changing your diet from day one of the program. If you are not interested in changing your diet to a healthier one by reducing or eliminating certain foods, you may not be a good fit for this type of program.

Many offices offer free workshops or open houses, or even videos on their website. If you can attend a workshop or open house this is a way to meet the doctor, learn what they know and see if their clinical programs might work for you.

Remember that most alternative practitioners work with therapies that are not covered by insurance. Many do not bill insurance at all, and most are cash practices. If you start your search by eliminating any provider who doesn't take your insurance, you will be severely reducing your choices.

For me, the most important things I require in a healthcare provider are care and clinical competence. I want to feel the doctor knows and understands me, listens to me and is invested in my health care and in getting results! You want a practice and a doctor who wants to get results for you, and who measures these results over time by repeating labs and seeing if you are achieving positive changes from the program you embark upon. It is important to have this quantitative objective testing to determine your progress, in addition to how you feel.

There is a way to have a healthy body. There is a way to resolve chronic health concerns. Death will come to all of us, but the question is how have we lived our lives? Who did we help? Did we live our passions and chase our dreams? Did we do those things that meant something to us? Did we have the health to be able to do these things? Can we look back and be proud of what we have accomplished and what we have left behind?

There have been times in this world when a prophet or other mystic would bring the miracles of healing to us and with the barest touch of their hand, raise the dead or heal the sick. The dramatic struggle for how to heal the human body is age old. From dances, sticks in the fire, potions and spells, sorcery and superstitions to the "magic drugs" and the surgeries of today, all of these have passed as solutions to the body's ills.

That faith alone could accomplish such things has engendered hope and sent many on journeys of discovery for a lifetime in search of healers and mystics. Many books and documentaries have been written about these mysteries. I would like to suggest that the type of true healing that I have spoken of in this book is not a belief or a religion or a miracle, unless we define the body's own healing as a miracle.

From experience with countless patients, I've seen that common sense, science and a knowledge of the human body can create many "modern day miracles" where only pain and death were foretold previously by conventional doctors. When a drug or surgery does nothing to fix a problem and when a person cannot be responsible in some way for their own health condition and has no action they could take to fix themselves, they are completely stuck. They must rely fully on someone or a system to "fix" them, and that system has no ability to do this. This is what we all know now as modern medicine.

I would like to propose a better way. We currently have a technology that systematically and successfully addresses common chronic health concerns. This technology enables your body to be well and empowers you to have the health you need to accomplish all the things you came into this world to do.

Let me help you find your healing. It is within each one of us. We have just to reach out to find it. You are here to make this world better. If I did not truly believe this, you would not be reading this book. Your passion, your love, your journey, your path will touch hundreds if not thousands of lives. You are my smart woman, my warrior princess, my fearless mom, my loving wife, student extraordinaire and star of your own life.

Like ripples in water, our lives, our choices and our decisions reach places we could never have imagined. For me, my health is a means to an end. If I am healthy and I can stand in front of you and help you find healing, we together can go out into a world that is hurting and offer strength and love and healing to others. We are here to make a difference, at home, at work, in the world at large, in big and small ways every day.

As women, we are a force to be reckoned with. If your force is a little low, let me encourage you and give you hope, because when you have hope, you have everything. Be the champion of your own world and your own story. Make the ending you want to your story and have the time of your life doing it! Let the symphony of your life play out beautifully for all to hear.

CHAPTER 15
Women Who Took Charge of Their Health

Here are the stories of some of my patients who range in age from their twenties to their seventies. They embody the smart women I wrote this book for. They exude determination and focus, and in looking for a way to regain their health naturally they found me. In working together, we took their own personal health care to a level that enabled them to find wellness again. As with most things, health is always a journey and not just a destination.

I have included these stories because I hope you see something of yourself in these women. They are the success stories in their own lives. They wrote their own symphony and it is beautiful! I love their thoughts and their strength. I love seeing their brilliance in overcoming the bumps of life and the lessons they learned as a result. Their stories bring me hope that we all can create the life and health that we want. They made the decisions, they made the life choices, and I was honored to serve as their coach and guide. I hope you enjoy their stories, transcribed below exactly as they told them to me, and I hope you are as inspired by these stories and by these women as I am!

Elise

Elise is determined, resourceful and talented. She is an actor and an artist, and a really smart woman. Even though she is young, she realized she needed help to get to the cause of her problems, as well as the resources necessary to make it all happen herself. Elise has my respect! This is her story.

> *When I started school, I remember having health issues. My mom said I didn't have any health problems as a baby, and she thought it had a lot to do with introducing processed foods in school lunches.*
>
> *My biggest problem was stomach cramps. I was six or seven years old and it was the most painful thing ever. I hated it. I would have these awful cramps and I'd be on the ground crying when I would*

have to go the bathroom. It was terrible. We thought it was lactose intolerance, because it seemed to happen when I ate ice cream. I just accepted it as normal.

As a teenager I didn't notice it as much, though I do remember sometimes being bloated. When I went to college, it started up all over again, even worse. I gained a lot of weight and I did drink alcohol. I was literally trying to find all kinds of supplements to help me. I went to health food stores. I went to yogi people. I asked lots of questions, looking for solutions. In my third year of college, I changed everything I ate. I moved off campus and started to cook my own food. That helped a lot. I lost fifteen pounds.

After college and learning what I should and should not eat, my health leveled out a bit. But my digestion was just not functioning right. I could take apple cider vinegar shots, or do a detox cleanser pill every single night, and it would work for a little while, then these would stop working and I would be back where I started again.

For three of the last four years, it got worse, to the point where I would be extremely bloated, and I wouldn't be hungry, so I just wouldn't eat. If I tried to eat I just felt awful. I had a very bad relationship with food, because it would always make me feel worse.

I was really bloated for multiple days, and I had gained fifteen pounds over the course of four years. The last year I was trying really hard to eat healthy, and I was working out constantly. I was getting frustrated. I went to a doctor who wanted to give me a pill. I was like, "I'm not going to be the person who is on pills for the rest of my life. I really think that you can heal your own body."

I believe in energy healing and I do believe in Reiki and acupuncture, but I feel like it's more than that. I feel like it's a process, a combination of things. I read your Evectics information and that process made a lot of sense to me. The idea makes sense to me and works with my belief system. That's how I landed in your lap!

I came to you and did the step-by-step program that you recommended for me. You gave it a name. That helped a lot. I felt like I wasn't doing trial and error any more. Giving me a plan and a process was really helpful. It was great! Whether it's environmental or genetic or whatever the cause is, I'd like to know what it is! It's got to be something right? I'm a why person, I like having the labs and reading them over. I like being able to have things tested and see what is wrong and know there is a way to resolve it.

There is so much information out there and you can go down the rabbit hole of researching and learning. I think that education is a really big thing. There are some things you read that flat out don't make sense if you know enough about how the body works. Knowing your body and knowing how things work is very helpful!

Now, I've gotten to the point where I don't always need afternoon coffee depending on how long my day is. Sometimes I don't need it in the morning either, if I had a really good night's sleep. I'm learning that I don't always have to strive for perfection in every little thing. I realize that some days are different than other days because of hormonal stuff. I think it is very important for women to realize this. We are different on different days of the month. I have learned that with me there's about one week of the month where I'm weird, I'm not a good human and I feel very tired. I do things differently to help myself during these times. I don't strive for perfection these days.

I'm an actress and I've worked in many different jobs. I've been aware of my health for a very long time. I do want to say that if we did more preventative care earlier as women we would not have to do so much restorative care. Your early twenties should be geared towards restorative and preventive care. It is completely worth it whatever you have to do to fix your health now. I would say to everybody, pay attention and learn about your body in your twenties or thirties, and fix the things that are wrong now, then you won't have issues in your fifties and sixties.

We're not meant to live with the stress we've given ourselves. So much of illness is stress. Understanding your thoughts, and the way you can give yourself anxiety issues is all tied in with health and healing and learning this early is good. I know that I'm going to have a lifetime of health maintenance, but I feel like that's the easier thing to do, now that I have found the things that work well for me. I shouldn't have any issues in my later life.

This program that I have done here is worth it. I have learned so much. I'm a much happier person when I feel healthy and I feel good. I can now put more positive energy into the things that I'm doing and want to do. There are a lot of things that I want to do, I can't be putting energy into my digestive system for the rest of my life. I need it to just work. I've done so well! I have had less bloating in the last three months than I have had in the last three years. It makes me feel good.

When I was in high school, I wanted to major in theatre. I loved theater, it was my favorite thing. I wasn't going to major in theatre in college, but I had this long-term substitute teacher and I told her I couldn't major in theater. She said, "Why not?" I literally hurt after that question. I realized I had no actual reason. Her asking me why not when I had no actual reason made me realize I didn't know why I was not going to major in theater when I loved it so much.

This one statement had a huge impact on my life. It made me examine what I was thinking. As a result, doing. I was sixteen or seventeen then, but now every time someone tells me that they can't do something, I ask, "Why not?" If I think I can't do something or someone tells me I can't do something, especially because I am a woman, I ask myself Why not? It's about not accepting things in your life that aren't working, and really examining your choices.

What you allow in your life is what the rest of your life will be shaped by, and complacency is one of the most frustrating things. I remember somebody told me, "You're getting older, that's just how it is," and I'm like "No, that's not how it is, that's ridiculous!"

That's the most absurd thing I've ever heard. I can absolutely find the problem and I can be as healthy as I want to be! Why not?

Kristen

Kristen is a lovely, determined and passionate advocate for health and healing. Here is her amazing story of how she found her health, and never gave up through some of the most difficult and dark times of her life.

I first started noticing health issues back in eighth grade. Ten to fifteen years ago people weren't really addressing autoimmune diseases. There's a history of those issues in my family. I couldn't really eat anything. I was really small, but I refused to eat because it would hurt.

In high school, I would be okay for a while and then I would get terrible bloating, gas and diarrhea. I self-diagnosed lactose intolerance. I've always been an athlete and been on different teams. I was a swimmer. Throughout the season, I noticed that I was getting lightheaded in the pool. I would have a hard time catching my breath and I would get kind of dizzy. We went to my doctor at the time, and she told me that I was overweight and that it was my cycle. She wanted to put me on medication. I didn't want to be on any medication.

The issues got worse throughout the year. My lightheadedness was getting severe. I started to black out when my heart rate went up. I had a few times where I would go for a run and have to turn around, because I was about to pass out. I had to lay down on the floor in front of the fan and drink juice. I couldn't go for a swim because every time I got my heart rate up I would start to black out.

I went to different doctors, starting with a general physician. He sent me to a cardiac specialist, who put me on some kind of medication. He did a test, and I passed out within the first twenty seconds. My heart rate dropped to 25 or 30, and my blood pressure tanked. They put me on a medication for vasovagal syncope. I tried this for a couple weeks. It wasn't working, but he upped the dosage. He gave me no other options. He wasn't exploring any other areas or causes.

I went to a neurologist next. He was different. He listened. He was attentive. He said, "The only thing I can think of is that your sister has migraines and maybe you have exercise-induced migraines, which can produce some of the side effects that you're talking about." He took me off the cardiac medicine and put me on a very strong migraine medication.

The medication started to work, and I was able to start exercising again. Because I couldn't exercise, I had put on weight. I was anxious and depressed. When I started to exercise again with this medication I started to lose some of the weight I had gained. Within a couple months, we had upped my dosage and I was taking about 400 mgs a day of this stuff. I started losing my word recall. I would try to say something that was on the tip of my tongue, but I just couldn't get it out. I lost thirty pounds in three months. I was very controlling and very restrictive with myself and my food, I was borderline eating disorder.

After high school, I wanted to travel with a mission to Honduras, Thailand, and South Africa. I was really concerned that I would not be able to get my medication while I was overseas, and I would have issues with the heat. My side effects were brought on by extreme heat and dehydration. We were at the training camp in Georgia. It was 100 degrees. They prayed over me and I decided to stop my medication. I had no side effects and I was able to do rigorous training and I felt good. I believe God really cures.

Traveling in Honduras, I had severe digestive issues, and after contracting bronchitis and pneumonia I received many rounds of antibiotics and steroids. These did resolve the infections but destroyed my gut further and I felt horrible. In Thailand, we ate a lot of fruit and rice. I got better there, and I was able to exercise a little bit. In South Africa, we were once again back to eating mostly carbs, and a lot of dairy. We weren't really allowed to go out and be super active. I got very sick again. By the time I returned home from that trip, I had gained thirty-five pounds. During this time, I was eating gluten and feeling very bad; tired, and achy. I decided to try a gluten-free diet, and I lost fifteen pounds in a month.

I moved to Georgia in the fall. I was working a very manual job at the time and I got sick a lot. If I ate any kind of gluten, I'd be out *for two days from work, because it wiped me out. My stomach had gotten so sensitive by this time, that eating almost anything upset it. I felt bad all the time. I was really inflamed, so after Christmas, I went on an elimination diet. I cut out dairy, gluten, alcohol, and sugar.*

I got better and lost the weight from the inflammation. When I came to Alternative Health Atlanta to do a program, I was eating so restrictively, and I didn't want to spend the rest of my life so limited in what I could eat. I did the Systems Desensitization Technique to enable me to eat more food items as I was avoiding so many things to keep from getting sick. I just wanted to be able to eat somewhat normally again. Even with the elimination diet, everything in my body was wiped out. My adrenals were under extreme stress, my thyroid was not functioning well, my cortisol levels were way off, my stomach and large intestine were inflamed, and my menstrual cycle was still a problem.

Getting on probiotics and digestive enzymes was very important for me. After doing my program at AHA and desensitizing the foods I was sensitive to, I was still hesitant to introduce any new foods back into my diet, because I knew how badly I had felt in the past when I would eat them. I really wanted to give my body time to heal. After two-and-a-half months on my program, we slowly brought some food items back in. My cycles normalized about three months in, and that was just one sign I was getting better.

Because of my program and my diet changes, I had my energy back. I could eat "normal" foods now without getting sick and I could work and have a life. I struggled for a long time and it was so good to have found answers and solutions to my health issues.

I am currently studying to be an herbalist. I want to help people become well in an affordable and accessible way. I want to empower people to lead their families into wellness. I want to educate people on how to raise their kids in a healthy way and what to do if their kids are sick like I was. I am thankful for my own journey because I know it will help me to help others that much more.

I would tell people who are struggling with these kinds of health issues that there is hope! Coming into a true partnership with your body is possible. Our bodies were designed to be cared for and treated with respect. Wellness is a journey and a commitment— one that is ours for a lifetime.

There will be setbacks along the way and frustrations, but that is okay. Those of us who have been sick for almost all our lives may believe that health is not in the cards for us, that somehow, we drew the short straw. THIS IS NOT TRUE! Believing that there is healing for you and becoming your own advocate is the step that makes the difference. You are worth the time it takes. You are worthy of finding answers to your long-ignored questions. There is healing for you. You are a beautiful human being created to be well and to live your life to its fullest potential. ALL bodies were created for fullness of life, including yours!

Paula

Paula's story is amazing! She found me in her later years after she raised her family and was at retirement age. She wants to be as healthy as she can be, to enjoy her family and her life. She does not want to be at the doctor every week suffering from chronic health problems and taking medications for all the things that ail her. She is a beautiful woman who is strong and smart, and is one of the moms and wives who stuck it out against tremendous odds to raise wonderful kids, create a home and a fulfilling career.

She knows her body can heal itself, and she was willing to make lifelong changes in her diet and lifestyle that will enable her to achieve her long-term health goals. The spirit that she and many of my female patients embody is a testament to the true grit and determination of the female spirit, and I celebrate this in all of us.

"I've been coming to Dr. Billiot now for about four months. I am happy to find that there's an option other than just medical doctors who only give me medication for the different issues that I've had over the years.

I, like a lot of women, have had a family to take care of. I raised four children, had a husband that I've been married to for forty-

eight years, and a full-time career in a male-dominated field. My goal was to be the best mother, the best wife, and the best and top employee of wherever I worked. That created a lot of stress. I just kept driving myself and driving myself to be the best at everything, to the point of exhaustion.

Unfortunately, it's difficult to keep all the balls in the air for a long, extended period, but I was striving to do so. During the 1980s, it was very important for women to try to be superwoman, to do it all: cook, have a career, raise a family, all those things. I had extreme amounts of stress. After about twenty-five years of trying to do my best to make sure everybody had everything they needed, the stress caught up with me. I did what most women typically do. We go until we cannot go anymore, we forget about ourselves.

My doctor one day said, "I want you to go home and get in the bed, and don't get out for at least a month." I'm thinking, How am I going to do that with a family, and a household to run? *I ended up being out of work for about five months, just recuperating, because I was so exhausted. I wish I would have known there were some other choices, like helping your body do what it's supposed to do and assisting it heal itself, instead of pushing it beyond its limits, and running on empty. I would have cherished the opportunity to have availed myself of the services that I have been doing here at your clinic for the last four months, back then as a younger me.*

During that time, it was like the movie Steel Magnolias. *We had to be those steel magnolias, just so we could do it all. When I was in my early twenties, I didn't feel equipped to be in one of the careers women were likely to go into, like nursing or being a secretary. I wanted to be in sales, because I love people and I liked being out and about. I didn't want to be fenced in, but my job was extremely stressful. In 1980, when I started, I was the first female in sales in Western Union. Of course, they wanted me to fail because I was entering their territory. I proved, however, that wasn't going to happen.*

I knew the sales district I was assigned was in the most dangerous part of Atlanta. When I would go on appointments, I would take my network engineer with me who was a male. We were designing data networks and changing the way people ran their businesses. When I arrived at a business, they didn't expect a young lady, a blonde, to be in technology. For them to believe me, I had to introduce him as my network engineer, and tell them that if I said anything incorrect he would speak up and correct me.

They sat there and listened to me only because he was there. It was a difficult time to forge new territory for women, because women were not generally in the technology field, but I did it anyway and became a top sales person.

It wore me out. I was trying to grasp the new technology, and it was evolving all along. As technology evolved, I was responsible for going out and introducing it to company headquarters throughout Georgia to change the way they'd been communicating with their vendors. I had to study every night. I would put my four children to bed, and then I would study, because the next day I had to go out and talk to somebody about something new that nobody had ever talked about before.

All the while, I was still trying to keep my husband happy because he liked to be active on the weekends, and we enjoyed traveling, and boating, and different things. We were also active in the children's lives, whatever activity they were involved in. There was never a moment to rest.

It's been an interesting journey, and a very rewarding one. I showed myself that I could do it, but I paid a price, health-wise. My weight's always been an issue for me. It goes up and down and I did every diet that came along. It would work for a little while and I'd feel good. Then I'd lose some pounds and it didn't take long to gain it right back. The only thing that ever worked for me was this program at Alternative Health Atlanta and Weight Watchers, because what works is teaching you to eat correctly, make better choices and make lifestyle changes that are important to long term health.

Now, I'm using the education and the techniques and tools that you have taught me here to assist my body to heal. I just am really thrilled that I have this program. With all the labs, and tests, I have more information on what's going on in my body than I ever have before. These tools, as well as the acupressure techniques that you use, have combined to help me get at the root of my health problems and get healthier inside. It's really been a total about-face.

From my perspective, people like myself are retiring and want to be healthy. I worked hard for what I have. I'm very appreciative of what I have done in my life, and humbled that the Lord's let me enjoy so much. I also don't want to spend my retirement going to the doctor. I don't want to spend what I have on a hospital bill and being laid up and unable to do what I want to do and go where I want to go.

I'm finally able to be without the huge responsibilities that I've had my whole life and I am ready to enjoy the world. I've been blessed to have gone to every continent on this planet, some of them two or three times. I can't continue to do this if I am not healthy enough. I want to go and see everything that I can. I want to see things that are far away, and experience places and lands that are dangerous, and rowdy while I still am able. I'm going to try to stay this way as long as I can. I don't want to spend my good hard-earned money on health issues. If I can be as healthy as my body will let me be and minimize these issues, I think that's a lot better way to go!

There's a huge difference between conventional and alternative medicine. There's no comparison. It's like night and day. A physician diagnoses whatever disease someone may have. Then they say, "We'll give you some medicine for it." It may or may not work, you never really know if it works or not. You just throw it in your body and hope that it will. Sometimes, maybe your blood pressure goes down, or your blood sugar goes down and you can see if those issues respond to the medication, but you don't ever get to the root cause of the problem.

In this clinic, the technology is always, always working at getting to the root cause of what the issue is. I like to get to the cause and find out what's going on inside of my body, which I can do with this program. Here, we don't mask symptoms with medicine just so we won't feel the pain or won't have the effect of the illness. I can be as healthy as I can be and by learning new habits, taking the exact supplements I need and eating right, and I won't have to have medicine. That's my goal.

It's all about making choices that are healthy, and that's been a real learning curve for me. Since I've been here, I have been doing some of those "right things". I've given up sweets, which is something tremendous that you helped me with. That was my real weakness. I haven't wanted a sweet since I started on this program and when you did the acupressure treatment for sugar cravings, it totally took away my cravings for sugar, which is a miracle. Nobody that knows me can believe it.

I love that my family's taking advantage of the programs here, and doing it at an early age, and not repeating my history. All the grandchildren are going to be raised healthier. It's just fabulous. It took me forever to discover and find this type of healthcare, so that my body can heal itself. I've lost twenty-three pounds so far. I look forward to losing some more. I am excited to see the many changes, with my blood sugar on the way to being normal and less medication for me! That's my goal. That will be awesome for sure and I can do it. Sometimes you just must be willing to look at something new and say, "Well, my old ideas weren't working so it's time to do something new." I have seen living proof of this working for me and my family!

Cypria

Cypria is an inspiring woman on a journey to master herself in all aspects. I have been honored to be part of this journey, and to help her find tools to achieve her goals. She is strong. She is smart. She is a fighter, and she never gives up until she reaches her goals! Here is her story.

As a kid, I was diagnosed with food allergies. In spring and fall, with pollen and things flowering, times were hard times for me growing up. I remember waking up in March or April, sneezing ten or fifteen times, then feeling so tired. I couldn't go back to bed because I had to go to school.

In high school, I was put on antihistamines, which helped with sneezing and itchy eyes and the scratchy throat, but made me even more tired. We tried allergy shots for four or five years, and that kind of helped. I had eczema which would flare up in the spring. In university, by October my hands were cracked and bleeding, and that made writing and typing hard.

I was taking cortisone and a tar-based ointment to deal with the symptoms, but no one tried to find the underlying issues. When I was twenty-four, I was put on high blood-pressure medication, but I was always able to function. I had a chronic foot infection that came back, following my cycle. No effort was put into figuring out why boils and blisters would pop up right before my period then turn into open sores for weeks.

Then I went to Mozambique. My health in Mozambique was good, and my seasonal allergies disappeared. I was living in a rural community; most things were grown organically. I was eating a lot of vegetables, beans and fruit and not much dairy. When I was in university, while doing my undergrad, I developed what I call the Elvis regimen—caffeine to keep you up, then alcohol to put you to bed. My parents instilled this work ethic, "You suffer today to live well tomorrow." I assumed that when life was hard, and I was so tired and did not have much ambition to get things done in school, it was because I wasn't putting in enough effort, not that something could actually be physically wrong with my body.

After leaving Mozambique, my weight started ballooning and I gained about thirty pounds. I've always had menstrual cramps, but these got worse the last two months I was in Mozambique. I took a cocktail of 600 milligrams of ibuprofen every three and a half hours for the first day and then after the first day I was fine. It allowed me to function for about five hours and then the hum of pain drained me of energy, and I'd just lay there. I wasn't really of use to myself or to anybody else during those days of the month.

I was not doing well at all during this time. If I had trouble getting up in the morning, or going to sleep at night, or if I had difficulty concentrating, I just chalked it all up to my laziness. What else could it have been? I think everybody likes to have a break to slack off or to take it a little easy. I just attributed my inability to do the things that I wanted to get done to me needing a "break". I thought it was a discipline issue, rather than a physical, or health issue. I was playing psychological games with myself to get myself up. I really believed that if my will was stronger, if my dedication to my studies were better, if I were more organized, if I were more disciplined, I wouldn't be struggling the way I was.

I could not have been more wrong, it turned out. But the thing was, I DID NOT KNOW ANY BETTER. I thought it was all me, all my own laziness and inability to motivate myself sufficiently.

Things turned around when I started working with Dr. Billiot and doing my own health program with her. First, I just felt better! I remember telling my mom, "I don't care what this is, I am really better!" I was able to sleep at night, and mornings weren't so terrible.

I got my hair analysis results and my other labs back, and for the first time I could see and understand and read a test that showed me that things were out of balance and my body was "off" physically. I had an explanation!

One issue that was affecting my body greatly was an excess of copper that led to trouble concentrating, depression, and emotional liability, which I just thought was kind of in my personality. I am Type A: I love hard, I hate harder. I have ups and downs, and I burst into tears easily. I could always find a reason to cry. Knowing that I wasn't entirely responsible for the way I was feeling was really, really liberating. My struggles were not because I wasn't good enough, or strong enough, or dedicated enough, or focused enough, but really because my body was struggling! I was sick physically.

One thing I realized as well about myself was that I found the idea of self-care to be uncomfortable. I thought of "self-care" as soft music and candles and a bath and maybe a good book, and that's just not me. Because of this, I just did not understand what my body needed and what type of self-care was necessary for my body to stay healthy. I started to think, if my body was a car, I would take it into the shop to get tuned up, and its oil changed. I realized I was nicer to my car than to myself! It was a life-changing moment.

I knew in my gut and I had been telling my soul for a long time that something was wrong. I didn't have the tools to prove that something really was wrong with my body physically, so I just kind of ignored it. I want to tell other women that if you don't feel like yourself and you think that you should just be doing better, or working harder, if you think life should be better but you can't get yourself better, there's probably something going wrong physically and you should find out what it is.

I have new ideas about self-care now. We should practice self-care in the true sense, not in the temporary sense that we see on TV or in the media. Develop good habits. Do things for yourself like sleep enough and eat healthy food and exercise but do this because it's going to make you more effective.

There are a lot of expectations on women today. Some expectations are external, but somehow, we've internalized them as well. For myself, I often try to achieve some arbitrary, sometimes unrealistic, standards that I have set for myself. We must ask ourselves why does this arbitrary standard exist? Why is it that, along with everything else I must do to please everyone else, I also have to achieve these personal internal arbitrary expectations that I have laid on myself? I am still working on this! We all need to. We need to be kinder to ourselves and often the first step is realizing these internal expectations we ourselves have placed there, so we can change them.

In regard to food, I'm happier when I eat. I'm more respectful when I eat. I'm more alert when I eat. I know these things. I feel like as women we have a lot of societal expectations put on us at a very early age about weight and body image. These ideas come from media, pictures, from our mothers, not even meaning to, but you grow up in a culture that expects certain things. I really hate those societal things that we live with! I think sometimes, not even consciously, I am aware that these are the scripts we tell ourselves in the background. It might not be in the front of our minds, but they definitely are in the background. Bringing them forward to examine them gives you power over them.

One of the big things that I told myself, ever since I was little, was that I had a treasonous body. My body and I were not friends, that relationship was always conflictual because I could not get it to do what I wanted it to do. As an example, I loved gymnastics growing up. I did a lot of it, but I was never particularly good. I would practice, and I would practice, and I would practice but there were certain things that were just harder to do physically for me. I had very strong legs, so I could do floor stuff, but my upper body was not as strong as my legs. Pulling myself up on the beam, no matter how hard I practiced, was still a struggle for me. I just didn't understand why I couldn't get my body to do the thing that I saw in my mind, I knew what it looked like, but I couldn't get it to physically accomplish the picture that I had in my mind. I have realized since then that it wasn't about me; that my body was strong in different ways and it was not purposely betraying me! But this was a thought process that I took with me into adulthood.

There is no reason why you can't have what you want. It might not come in the form you think it's going to come in, but you can have everything you want. I never thought mastering my "treasonous" body and looking after my health would be the first step to doing that. In looking after my health, I've also started to dismantle that idea of my body being treasonous. I have the tools now. I've finally gotten to the point where I understand enough about my body so that I can get my body to do what I want and need it to do and I am willing to do the things necessary to help it achieve this state. It is a good place. I'm also at a point now where I realize that maybe the things I wanted to do in the past aren't the best or the healthiest. I guess I could still be a psycho person and keep exercising and working out in a crazy unhealthy way to get to be that size two, punishing my "bad body" to achieve this "goal" or maybe this is not really what I want. Maybe with good sensible self-care, my body could be trained to do something that would enable me to be healthier and happier and more myself.

I would tell people, "You do deserve to have those things that are for your best good and for your highest good, and it's okay to let go of the things that you figure out are not as beneficial." I would tell other women, "You deserve to be effective at fulfilling your purpose, because ultimately that's my definition of happiness." A lot of times people are trying to get a job done, or stay in a relationship, or get through school, and their bodies are sort of betraying them, because they're not healthy. They haven't taken the time to even see whether there is a problem, and whether there is something that can be done about it. People don't take the time to make sure they are sleeping, make sure they've got the right food. They do not make sure they have a stress level their lives can maintain, they do not have stability and balance. I think these are the things you must have as a prerequisite for almost anything you want to accomplish.

Do your research. Find a health program that will work for you. Find something that will resonate with you. Being healthy or getting on the road to health is a process like anything else. It's about being mindful and living in the moment. Take your supplements and learn to be healthy! I did. You can too.

Aubrey

Aubrey is a yoga teacher, a missionary, a dance instructor, and an overall fantastic woman. She has faced a health journey that contained some real challenges to her and to her future. She met these with determination and incredible results for her health. It wasn't always easy, and Aubrey has traveled from out of town to my office to stay on her health program despite many obstacles, including distance, time and money. I have been so proud of her and so in awe of her determination to be well. Literally nothing gets in her way. Aubrey gives much to the world, and I cannot wait to see where her story leads her.

The pressure is immense. The expectation on young women today is to have a successful career, a picture-perfect husband and kids, and to be a Pinterest-worthy mother who still has time to make that afternoon yoga class followed by a healthy green smoothie, and then afford a trip to the organic aisle of Whole Foods. In all the chaos, we fall for self-help tips instead of getting to the root of why we need them in the first place. As a culture, we have lost the value of rest and jumped on the hamster wheel of productivity at the expense of our health.

I have had health problems since as long as I can remember, starting as a severely colicky baby to chronic digestive problems, headaches, fatigue and back pain most of my childhood. I literally dragged myself through the day in high school and took a hot shower every morning to combat the severe headache I woke up with each day. I lived a jam-packed lifestyle and used food mostly as a comfort or a remedy for stress.

By the time I was a freshman in college it all began to take its toll. I was struggling to have the energy to keep up with life's demands, and spent a lot of time sick in bed. I lost friendships because I couldn't spend time with friends, let alone do my school work and work my job. And forget trying to exercise! I felt like I was wasting away and on a slippery slope.

To top it all off, my symptoms went from chronically frustrating to scary and serious. I began developing breast cysts and severe migraines. I would pass out in heat or if my heart rate went up at all. I was losing my memory and my brain was foggy all the time. I was anxious and depressed and on an emotional roller coaster. My menstrual cycles were unbearable and left me dead to the world for three to five days. At this point in my life, I had seen almost every kind of doctor with an "ologist" at the end of their name. They offered me no hope and left me so discouraged.

I decided to stop eating gluten and saw a huge improvement in my symptoms. I was able to finish college. However, a year into my marriage, I realized that although I was functional, the things I was fighting with daily were not normal and were certainly not sustainable. I couldn't fathom starting a family while I was still fighting to get through each day.

This was my story until I met Dr. Billiot, which was a true answer to a prayer my husband and I had prayed. In a few hours she was able to answer the laundry list of questions I had about my health problems and was the first doctor to address the many weird, seemingly unrelated health issues that were impairing my quality of life. It was such a relief but for me it was also so hard to believe. After spending my whole life having well respected doctors tell me that there is nothing wrong with me and that nothing could be done, really took a toll on my outlook. I had believed them, and it took some convincing labs and lots of discussion for me to see how sick my body really was and that there was hope for me.

It wasn't an easy journey to healing. I truly had to reevaluate my priorities and realize what was most important to me. Was I willing to make some sacrifices to have a healthier life? I had to pick and choose where to spend my time and energy so that I could have the lifestyle that I truly wanted, one with time for family and friends, one with boundaries and rest, and most importantly one in which I was healthy. As I began to make some very needed life changes, some easy and some very hard to choose, I began to truly enjoy my life. I had time to sleep and rest, time to eat right and enjoy cooking my food.

I remember one instance in which I went home from a treatment and as I drove home I began to feel this warmth spread through my body, my abdomen and my back (weird sounding I know). By the time I got home I told my husband, "This is so weird, but I feel like someone is giving my insides a hug." I thought about it and then it dawned on me... what I was feeling for the first time in my life was the absence of pain! I had no idea that I was living with so much discomfort because I hadn't known anything different.

As I continued following my program my anxiety and worry began to dissipate, and my blood sugar problems went away as I committed myself to healthy living and to the treatment program at AHA. I began to understand that life wasn't about having it all but enjoying what I did have and knowing how to value what was most important. I had to change more than just foods to have the lifestyle and health that I wanted, but it was well worth it, and a tribute to the patience and contributions of Dr. Billiot and the staff at AHA."

Alicia

Alicia and I met twenty years ago, when I had just started my practice. My oldest son was not even born yet.

When I met Alicia at a talk I was giving at a health club, she was my volunteer who came up to the front of the group to have muscle reflex testing demonstrated on her. When I tested her, I found several reflexes that indicated that she might be having some problems with blood sugar between meals. Her reaction was something she and I will never forget! She accused me and the health club manager of having spoken about her previously for me to have known this! Of course, this was the first time I had met either of them.

We helped her body fix her life-long blood sugar problems and from that day on, Alicia realized she had found a place to help her body help itself.

Over the course of the twenty years she has worked with me, we have addressed any and all things that have arisen health-wise and age-wise for her. We have given her body an increased ability to heal itself and to get well. Alicia is on no medications, she travels and continues to work sometimes extremely long hours even in retirement, and has the energy and health of a much younger woman. She is a shining example of what can happen if you do the things necessary over a lifetime to keep your body and hormones healthy. Alicia has been a professional woman her whole life and I am so proud of the fact that she is willing to do every day what she needs to do to keep her health in tip top shape!

> *I met Dr. Billiot twenty years ago, when I was in my early fifties. I have been seeing her ever since. I am in excellent health and I consider that one of the major contributing factors to this is Dr. Billiot's practice.*
>
> *I firmly believe that the human body can heal itself, and this is what her practice is all about. I don't take any prescription drugs or over-the-counter medications because I believe that the human body does not need them, and that they do more harm than good. I believe that the nutrition supplements Dr. Billiot has recommended for me over the years have helped to maintain my good health."*

Martha

Martha is a brilliant woman who travels the world hiking and walking miles with the "young ones" she travels with. She is a professional woman in her late sixties who even now works full time as a flight attendant and a philanthropist for several charities. She takes no prescription meds, and is one smart lady. I met Martha about nine years ago when she came to my office trying to solve a chronic health problem. Over the years she has learned much about her health and her body, and working with her has taught me much as well.

"About nine years ago I had a chronic, severe cough, twenty-four hours a day, for more than a year. Two MDs diagnosed bronchitis and prescribed inhalers and antihistamine pills. I took the medication for about a month with no dramatic improvement and decided at sixty years of age I was not going to do this the rest of my life.

I was in Bombay, India and went to a clinic for a facial and had reflexology for the first time. I told the reflexologist that I had lung issues. I found the reflexology treatment interesting. That night I went to the airport to travel home. I could not believe that my cough stopped. I decided that when I got home I was going to search for a reflexologist. My cough returned in about a week.

An acquaintance had talked about seeing Dr. Billiot and being happy with the outcome. I assumed Dr. Billiot would have a reflexologist on staff or be able to recommend one. I went to her office, asked at the desk if they could recommend a reflexologist. They said they could not. I thanked them, and left. On my way to my car, a woman approached me and introduced herself as Dr. Billiot. She asked me what I was looking for. (She'd overheard my conversation in the office and had followed me out to see if she could answer any questions.)

I told her about my cough and she said she thought she could help me. She was able to squeeze me into her schedule that afternoon (at my request) and examined me. She explained that all my cleansing organs were overwhelmed with debris created by immune system challenges and that we would need to do some labs and other tests to find out exactly which ones. My sinuses were draining, causing my cough.

She recommended some specific supplements and told me to not eat sugar or anything that turns to sugar easily. I told her that could be a problem because I have had a glass of red wine daily much of my adult life. But I did what she told me. That was on Thursday afternoon. By Saturday afternoon, my coughing had been reduced by at least 75%. I couldn't believe the coincidence and then thought perhaps Dr. Billiot was onto something. I had spent years and a lot of money going to medical doctors who prescribed drugs that never worked, ever, and in two days my cough was 75% improved! WOW!

I went for my follow-up appointment on Monday. I told her I couldn't believe my cough had diminished so much. She nodded, smiled and kept testing me. Her assistant then proceeded to do the Systems Desensitization Technique therapy with me to desensitize some of the items my body was sensitive to. I followed her instructions. When we were finished she asked if I felt okay. I said yes and wondered what the "tapping" on the acupuncture points was all about. Dr. Billiot came in and asked how I felt. I looked her in the eye, told her, "This is the weirdest place I have ever been, but I would do whatever you told me to do because you are the only person who has been able to help me with my cough!"

For one year, I took all my supplements, did not eat sugar or drink alcohol, maintained a good diet and visited Dr. Billiot on a regular basis. I was not overweight but lost ten pounds. Various medical tests, lab tests and Dr. Billiot's testing indicated I was much healthier one year later. My cough was 90% gone.

I have learned many things but one of the most important is that when we are sick, we need to discover the root of our illness (areas of our body that need to be strengthened) and help our bodies to become stronger and to work more efficiently so our body itself can repair or cure what ails us. God designed our body to repair itself and to heal.

It is very apparent to me that much of the medications prescribed only mask symptoms, and do not repair the body. In fact, medication can cause additional problems in the body. I remember when this became so clear to me. A friend asked me if Dr. Billiot cures high blood pressure. I asked Dr. Billiot the same question and she replied, "That's not the right question."

She explained that high blood pressure is a symptom indicating something in the body is creating the high pressure and the body must get oxygen to the tissues. If it cannot, this can be one reason why the pressure will rise.

She said it was best to determine what might be creating stress in the body and to help the body heal. Finding out what was wrong and helping the body to overcome those obstacles could be very beneficial to my overall health.

I went home and thought about that. Next time I saw her I told her I was thinking that if I went to a conventional doctor for high blood pressure and was prescribed high blood-pressure medication, could this somehow mask the symptom of the high blood pressure and never address the underlying cause? I wondered if the medication lowering my blood pressure might be fighting with my body which was raising my blood pressure for reasons never discovered. She said yes, that could happen. That exchange really clarified in my mind how much modern medicine treats symptoms and not causes of illness.

Medications can be necessary, but I want to always know what the cause of my problem is. I know when I come to Dr. Billiot that is what we will be doing, looking for the underlying cause and doing those things that make my body stronger and more able to handle whatever stress life throws at me.

It becomes clear to anyone who interacts with her that Dr. Billiot is a brilliant scientist. That, combined with her amazing artistry with the human body, is beautiful to observe. Her innovative approach to health will dramatically change this country. I feel that her approach will revolutionize health, economics and government."

Yvette

I was beside myself with joy from my lab results! I am sure you see this all of the time but I thought them to be extraordinary, particularly to be where I am now from where I came in such a short time.

I knew I was not well, Dr. Billiot and I had known this for some time. I felt my family needed me and I thought if I kept my weight down, ate right, exercised, and supplemented my diet with quality products, I would be as good as I could be. However, I knew something just wasn't right, and secretly I carried around baby aspirin just in case that which I feared caught up with me.

I thought it was inevitable because my mother died from cardiovascular disease and so did my sister—both while under doctors' care and in the hospital for treatment or after release.

As I shared with you, I had resigned myself because I thought I already was doing what I needed to do. I didn't drink, I didn't smoke, I was right at or close to my ideal weight and I was active. I have a strong faith and just asked God to be with me. He was, and allowed me to do what I needed to do for my family in their worst moments and during their most needy times. He was there when you refused to update my supplements without my coming in. A godsend.

Three months ago, my blood pressure was at emergency levels, my total cholesterol level was over 300 my LDL level was close to 200. I was in a very bad place. I decided I had to change and change dramatically. I did what you recommended, and as a result my total cholesterol is 189 and my LDL is 79! That is a 150 point drop! My blood pressure is consistently in normal ranges now, without medication. It is nothing short of miraculous!

I now know what my future diet and exercise levels should be and with your help, I intend to be around for a very long time to come!"

All of us struggle. All of us have faults. We fail, we make mistakes, we cry and we learn. You are good enough, in fact you are better than good enough! As you are right now. Sometimes it is hard to see the important things for all the debris flying around, but what is important is you; your dreams, your goals, your laughter and your love. Strive to make these things your focus and be well. Create art, create beauty, create a better world right where you are. Be fierce! Be beautiful! Be you!

I wish you all healthy hormones and a long life of energy, focus and vitality!

Glossary

HORMONE Any of various chemical substances produced by body cells and released especially into the blood and having a specific effect on cells or organs of the body usually at a distance from the place of origin.

Also, a synthetic substance that acts like a hormone.

OVARY One of the usually two organs in the body of a female in which an egg (ovum) is produced.

UTERUS The organ of a female in which a baby develops before birth.

FALLOPIAN TUBE Either of a pair of tubes that carry an egg from the ovary to the uterus.

OVULATION The discharge of a mature ovum (egg) from the ovary—this is the time that a female human can become pregnant

OVARIAN FOLLICLES Fluid-filled sacs on the ovary containing an egg or ovum, released at ovulation

PROGESTERONE Progesterone is produced after ovulation by the corpus luteum (sack that the egg comes from) and is the hormone of the second half of the female cycle (luteal phase). Progesterone's main job is to control the buildup of the uterine lining and help mature and maintain this lining if there is a pregnancy. If there is no pregnancy, the progesterone levels fall, and the lining of the uterus is shed, which begins the menstrual cycle. Progesterone also helps to balance the effects of estrogen. Progesterone is known as the calming hormone.

ESTROGEN Estrogen is responsible for growing and maturing the characteristics of the female body and the reproduction system. Estrogen is produced mostly by the ovaries but also in smaller amounts by the adrenal glands and our fat cells. It regulates the first half of the menstrual cycle (follicular phase). Estrogen is referred to as the "growing hormone".

FOLLICLE STIMULATING HORMONE (FSH) This hormone is released from the pituitary gland in the brain. It is responsible for stimulating the ovarian follicles (fluid-filled sacs on the ovary containing an egg or ovum) to mature.

LUTEINIZING HORMONE (LH) This hormone is released from the pituitary gland in the brain at ovulation, and causes the rupture of the mature ovarian follicle, releasing the egg.

TESTOSTERONE A male hormone produced by the male testes that causes the development of the male reproductive system and the male sex characteristics. Testosterone is a very important sex hormone for both men and women, although women have much lower levels. This hormone is produced by the ovaries and adrenal glands (right on top of the kidneys). Testosterone helps women maintain muscle mass and bone strength. It enhances sex drive, and helps with an overall sense of well-being and zest for life.

MENSTRUATION The usually monthly bleeding and elimination of blood and tissue from the uterus that occurs in a female body from puberty to menopause.

HORMONE RECEPTOR A cell protein that binds a specific hormone. The hormone receptor may be on the surface of the cell or inside the cell. Many changes take place in a cell after a hormone binds to its receptor.

ENZYME A substance produced by a living organism that acts as a catalyst to bring about a specific biochemical reaction.

Acknowledgments

I want to acknowledge all the women in my practice whose lives I have touched and who have touched mine. You taught me as I taught you. You allowed me to help you and in doing so, have helped me more than I can easily say, and for that I am forever grateful. This book is for all the women who fight and live and work and breathe and give everything they have to their goals. You are my heroes and the people for whom I wrote this book. Be well. Be strong and know that there are answers to the questions you seek.

Love and acknowledgments to my grandma, Mary Hopkins Siple, who will be ninety-seven this December. She has always been my biggest fan and most importantly my friend! What a lucky girl I have been to have you in my life!

Much love to my Aunt Martha who motivated me and encouraged me to take the steps to write this book. I remember the day I decided it was time. You have believed in me and made me realize that I can change things in this world.

Thank you, Yvette, who came from the place of magic to be there at the right time to encourage and love me and to help me finish my work.

To my coach, Lynda Goldman, thank you from the bottom of my heart for motivating me to write this book and for reminding me of all the women who need to hear my voice and my message. You helped me get my book out of my head and into the hands of the women who need it most. Your art graces the cover of my book and your brilliance graces the world in the work that you do to help wellness authors give flight to their books and ideas.

Many thanks to my editors, Helen Wilkie and Norman Lowrey, and to my proofreaders Aubrey, Yvette and Gwen Kahn. All great books need great editors! I have the best!

A special thanks to Kristie Lynn from Archangel. Thank you so very much! My cover is gorgeous and you are an agel!

Thank you to Cheryl Chapman RN, HNC, for her life's work in women's breast health, for speaking with me, and for sharing her *phluffing the girls* with all of us!

Many thanks to Jeannette Encinias. Your poem, "Beneath the Sweater and the Skin" touched me so strongly that I knew I needed to share it with the people who would read this book. The emotion and the love you communicate is so powerful. I can feel my own Queen Owl wings beating beneath my sweater, and I thank you for this work of beauty reminding us all where true beauty lies.

To my special ladies who shared their stories for this book so that we may all learn from their experiences. I am so grateful and thankful for you all, Paula, Kristen, Yvette, Aubrey, Elise, Alicia, Cypria and Martha! A big acknowledgment to Alec Lowrey for the many hours spent transcribing these stories. Thank you as well to Lori Hamilton, Dr. Stewart Edrich, Nina Rae, Nelli Biddix, Michael Wisner, Stephanie Clement, Cheryl Chapman, Aubrey Van Benthem and Yvette Cologne for their time and early reviews of this book.

Many thanks and gratitude to you all!

– Dr. Billiot

About the Author

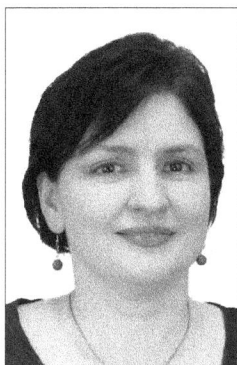

Dr. Melodie M. Billiot is the founder and owner of Alternative Health Atlanta, Holistic Practice Solutions (a company that develops techniques and management systems for holistic practitioners) and is the developer of the Evectics^{SM} health therapy systems.

She is known nationwide as an expert and sought-after teacher of nutritional and energetic techniques.

Dr. Billiot graduated from Life University in 1993 summa cum laude as valedictorian of her class. She is certified in CRA and Nutrition Response Testing, System Desensitization Technique (SDT) and N.A.E.T. allergy elimination techniques, System Balancing Technique (SBT), JMT, and several chiropractic adjusting techniques. She has also studied extensively in homeopathy, herbology, Chinese medicine, clinical nutrition and pain control using nutrition.

In 1994, she became frustrated because of a lack of consistent results with chiropractic treatment in areas other than musculoskeletal. Motivated to find a solution for her patients other than drugs and surgery, and fighting a serious health problem of her own, she started researching holistic and nutritional techniques. Because of this research, Dr. Billiot recovered her own health and made significant improvements in her results with patients.

Currently, Dr. Billiot has one of the most successful holistic practices in the country, and trains other practitioners in clinical nutrition and other holistic techniques.

She lives in Marietta, Georgia with her husband, their two boys, two dogs and two cats.

Join Us for Better Health!

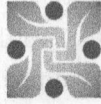

For more information and education on hormone health problems, or to learn about treatment options with my clinic, I invite you to join me at AlternativeHealthAtlanta.com.

If you're a health practictioner who would like to know more about our Evectics training programs, please contact me at:

DrMBilliot@AlternativeHealthAtlanta.com

Please Leave a Review

Thank you for reading this book. I hope you enjoyed it, and are starting the process of recovering your health.

Now I'd like to ask you for a small favor. Would you kindly take a moment to leave a review on Amazon? Here's a link to make it easier for you:

AlternativeHealthAtlanta.com/HarmonyReview

It would mean the world to me, and I am grateful for the time you take to write it!

Warmly,

Dr. Billiot

www.ingramcontent.com/pod-product-compliance
Lightning Source LLC
Chambersburg PA
CBHW050116280326
41933CB00010B/1125